ABC of
Sports and Exercise Medicine

Fourth Edition

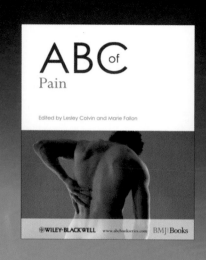
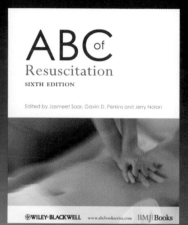
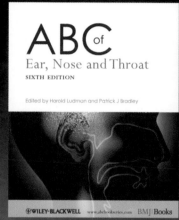
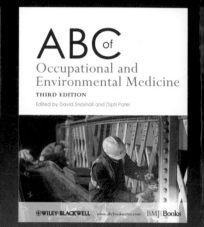
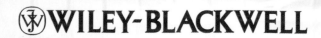

ABC of

Sports and Exercise Medicine

Fourth Edition

EDITED BY

Greg P. Whyte

Professor of Applied Sport & Exercise Science
Research Institute for Sport and Exercise Science
Liverpool John Moores University
Liverpool
UK

Mike Loosemore

Physician, English Institute of Sport
The Institute of Sport, Exercise and Health
University College London
London
UK

Clyde Williams

Professor of Sport Science
School of Sport, Exercise and Health Sciences
Loughborough University
Loughborough
UK

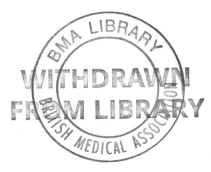

WILEY Blackwell

BMJ|Books

BMJ Books is an imprint of BMJ Publishing Group Limited, used under licence by John Wiley & Sons.

Registered office: John Wiley & Sons, Ltd, The Atrium, Southern Gate, Chichester, West Sussex, PO19 8SQ, UK

Editorial offices: 9600 Garsington Road, Oxford, OX4 2DQ, UK

The Atrium, Southern Gate, Chichester, West Sussex, PO19 8SQ, UK

111 River Street, Hoboken, NJ 07030-5774, USA

For details of our global editorial offices, for customer services and for information about how to apply for permission to reuse the copyright material in this book please see our website at www.wiley.com/wiley-blackwell

Library of Congress Cataloging-in-Publication Data

ABC of sports and exercise medicine / edited by Greg P. Whyte, Mike Loosemore, Clyde Williams.–4e.
    p. ; cm.–(ABC series)
Includes bibliographical references and index.
ISBN 978-1-118-77752-7 (pbk.)
I. Whyte, Gregory P., editor. II. Loosemore, Mike, editor. III. Williams, Clyde, editor. IV. Series: ABC series (Malden, Mass.)
[DNLM: 1. Sports Medicine. 2. Athletic Injuries. 3. Exercise. QT 261]
RC1210
617.1′027–dc23

2015015319

A catalogue record for this book is available from the British Library.

Wiley also publishes its books in a variety of electronic formats. Some content that appears in print may not be available in electronic books.

Typeset in 9.25/12pt MinionPro by SPi Global, Chennai, India

Printed and bound in Singapore by Markono Print Media Pte Ltd

1   2015

Contents

List of Contributors, vii

PART I   INJURY

1 Epidemiology of Sports Injuries and Illnesses, 1
Debbie Palmer-Green

2 Immediate Care in Sport, 5
Andy Smith

3 Head Injuries in Sport, 10
Daniel G. Healy

4 Injury of the Face and Jaw, 21
Keith R. Postlethwaite

5 Eye Injuries in Sport, 26
Caroline J. MacEwen

6 Management of Injuries in Children, 31
Julian Redhead

7 Management of Musculoskeletal Injuries in the Mature Athlete, 38
Khan Karim and Peter D. Brukner

8 Medical Care at Major Sporting Events, 41
Mike Loosemore

PART II   SYSTEM SPORT AND EXERCISE MEDICINE

9 Pulmonary Dysfunction in Athletes, 44
John Dickinson and James Hull

10 Infections, 50
Michael J. Martin

11 The Unexplained Underperformance Syndrome (Overtraining Syndrome), 54
Richard Budgett and Yorck Olaf Schumacher

12 The Female Athlete Triad, 58
Noel Pollock

13 The Athlete's Heart, 62
Aneil Malhotra, Greg P. Whyte and Sanjay Sharma

PART III ENVIRONMENTAL SPORT AND EXERCISE MEDICINE

14 Extreme Temperature Sport and Exercise Medicine, 67
Michael J. Tipton

15 Diving Medicine, 76
Peter T. Wilmshurst

16 Altitude Medicine, 81
Sundeep Dhillon

PART IV SPECIAL POPULATIONS

17 Physical Activity and Exercise as Medicine, 86
John Buckley

18 Sport, Exercise and Disability, 89
Nick Webborn

19 Sport, Exercise and Obesity, 93
David Haslam

20 Sport and Children, 97
Neil Armstrong

21 Physical Activity and Exercise in Later Life, 102
Dawn A. Skelton and Finbarr C. Martin

PART V NUTRITION AND DOPING

22 Nutrition, Energy Metabolism and Ergogenic Supplements, 109
Clyde Williams

23 Drugs in Sport, 116
Roger Palfreeman

24 Psychology of Injury, 122
Andrew M. Lane

Index, 127

List of Contributors

Neil Armstrong
Professor of Paediatric Physiology, Children's Health and Exercise Research Centre, University of Exeter, Exeter, UK

Peter Brukner
Consultant in Sport and Exercise Medicine, Olympic Park Sports Medicine Centre, Olympic Park, Melbourne, Australia

John Buckley
Professor of Applied Exercise Science, Institute of Medicine, University Centre Shrewsbury and University of Chester, UK

Richard Budgett
Medical and Scientific Director, International Olympic Committee, Lausanne, Switzerland

Sundeep Dhillon
Centre for Aviation Space & Extreme Environment Medicine, University College London, London, UK

John Dickinson
Senior Lecturer, University of Kent, Chatham Maritime, UK

David Haslam
Clinical Director, National Obesity Forum, Luton and Dunstable NHS Trust, Dunstable Road, Luton, UK

Daniel G. Healy
Professor of Neurology, Royal College of Surgeons, Ireland
Consultant Neurologist, National Neuroscience Centre, Beaumont hospital, Dublin, Ireland

James Hull
Consultant Chest Physician, The Royal Brompton Hospital, London, UK

Khan Karim
Consultant in Sport and Exercise Medicine, Qatar National Orthopedic and Sports medicine Hospital (ASPETAR), Doha, Qatar

Andrew M. Lane
Professor of Sport and Learning, Institute of Sport, Faculty of Education, Health and Well-being, University of Wolverhampton, Wolverhampton, UK

Mike Loosemore
Lead Consultant Sports Physician, English Institute of Sport, London, UK
The Institute of Sport, Exercise and Health, University College London, London, UK

Caroline J. MacEwen
Honorary Professor of Ophthalmology, University of Dundee, Dundee, UK

Aneil Malhotra
Department of Cardiology, St. George's Hospital Medical School, London, UK

Finbar C. Martin
Consultant Geriatrician at Guys & St Thomas' NHS Foundation Trust, London, UK
Hon. Professor of Medical Gerontology, Department of Ageing and Health, King's College London, GSTFT, St Thomas' Hospital, Westminster Bridge Road, London, UK

Michael J. Martin
Consultant Microbiologist, Royal Bournemouth Hospital, Bournemouth, UK

Roger Palfreeman
Consultant in Sport and Exercise Medicine, Claremont Hospital, Sheffield, UK

Debbie Palmer-Green
Senior Research Fellow, Arthritis Research UK, Centre for Sport, Exercise & Osteoarthritis, University of Nottingham, Nottingham, UK

Noel Pollock
Consultant in Sport & Exercise Medicine, Team Doctor British Athletics, London, UK

Keith R. Postlethwaite
Consultant Maxillofacial Surgeon, Newcastle upon Tyne NHS Hospitals Trust, Newcastle upon Tyne, UK

Julian Redhead
Consultant in Emergency Medicine, Imperial College School of Medicine, London, UK

Yorck Olaf Schumacher
Aspetar Orthopedic and Sports Medicine Hospital, Doha, Qatar

Sanjay Sharma

Consultant Cardiologist, Department of Cardiology, St. George's Hospital Medical School, London, UK

Dawn A. Skelton

Professor of Ageing and Health, School of Health and Life Sciences, Institute of Allied Health Research, Glasgow Caledonian University, Glasgow, UK

Andy Smith

Emergency Medicine Consultant Mid Yorkshire Hospitals NHS Trust, Wakefield, England

Yorkshire Ambulance Service BASICS Doctor, England

RFU Immediate Care in Sport Programme Director, Rugby Football Union, Twickenham, England

World Rugby Immediate Care in Rugby Technical Director and Senior Medical Educator, World Rugby, Dublin, Ireland

Michael J. Tipton

Professor of Human and Applied Physiology, Extreme Environments Laboratory, Department of Sport and Exercise Science, University of Portsmouth, Portsmouth, UK

Nick Webborn

Medical Director, Centre for Sport and Exercise Science and Medicine (SESAME), University of Brighton, Eastbourne, East Sussex, UK

Greg P. Whyte

Professor of Applied Sport & Exercise Science, Research intitute for Sport and Exercise Science, Liverpool John Moores University, Liverpool, UK

Clyde Williams

Professor of Sport Science, School of Sport, Exercise and Health Sciences, Loughborough University, Loughborough, UK

Peter T. Wilmshurst

Consultant Cardiologist, University Hospital of North Midlands, Stoke-on-Trent, UK

CHAPTER 1

Epidemiology of Sports Injuries and Illnesses

Debbie Palmer-Green

Senior Research Fellow, Arthritis Research UK, Centre for Sport, Exercise & Osteoarthritis, University of Nottingham, Nottingham, UK

OVERVIEW

- Sports injury and illness epidemiology research is continuing to grow
- Study design and methods can influence the conclusions made
- The definition of injury/illness, and rate and severity indices should be appropriate to the cohort of interest
- Identifying injury and illness causes will help to provide additional risk information
- Prevention initiatives should target the injury/illness issues posing the greatest risk

---

Introduction

Recognition of the importance of sports injury and illness epidemiology research has grown in the last 10 years with national and international governing bodies of sport regularly conducting surveillance at major sporting events. Most sports involve some element of risk with regard to athlete injury or illness, some significantly more so than other (Table 1.1).

Although much of the literature is focused on rehabilitation of athlete injuries (and illnesses), it is just as important to try and prevent them from occurring, or if it is not possible to prevent them completely at least lessen the severity and impact when injuries and illnesses do occur. In order to correctly prioritise and accurately target prevention initiatives to reduce injuries and illnesses in sport, it is important to understand the magnitude of the problem, that is, the rate and severity, and the causes. Conducting systematic monitoring of athlete injuries and illnesses in sport is essential to provide the evidence base to inform these prevention strategies. In order to get accurate and reliable data epidemiological study designs must be robust, and issues related to the design and implementation of injury and illness surveillance studies are discussed later, with illustrative examples provided.

Table 1.1 Rates of overall injuries and illnesses in the Olympic sports

Sport	No. of athletes	No. of injuries (%)	No. of illnesses (%)
Archery	128	2 (1.6)	10 (7.8)
Athletics	2079	368 (17.7)	219 (10.5)
Diving	136	11 (8.1)	7 (5.1)
Swimming	931	50 (5.4)	68 (7.3)
Synchronised swimming	104	14 (13.5)	13 (12.5)
Water polo	260	34 (13.1)	21 (8.1)
Badminton	164	26 (15.9)	5 (3.0)
Basketball	287	32 (11.1)	9 (3.1)
Beach volleyball	96	12 (12.5)	18 (18.8)
Boxing	283	26 (9.2)	18 (6.4)
Canoe slalom	83	2 (2.4)	4 (4.8)
Canoe sprint	749	7 (2.8)	14 (5.6)
BMX	48	15 (31.3)	2 (4.2)
MTB	76	16 (21.1)	5 (6.6)
Road cycling	210	19 (9.0)	7 (3.3)
Track cycling	167	5 (3.0)	16 (9.6)
Equestrian	199	9 (4.5)	11 (5.5)
Fencing	246	23 (9.3)	13 (5.3)
Football	509	179 (35.2)	62 (12.2)
Artistic gymnastics	195	15 (7.7)	5 (2.6)
Rhythmic gymnastics	96	7 (7.3)	1 (1.0)
Trampoline	32	2 (6.3)	1 (3.1)
Handball	349	76 (21.8)	17 (4.9)
Hockey	388	66 (17.0)	29 (7.5)
Judo	383	47 (12.3)	16 (4.2)
Modern pentathlon	72	6 (8.3)	1 (1.4)
Rowing	549	18 (3.3)	40 (7.3)
Sailing	380	56 (14.7)	38 (10.0)
Shooting	390	15 (3.8)	17 (4.4)
Table tennis	174	11 (6.3)	12 (6.9)
Taekwondo	128	50 (39.1)	14 (10.9)
Tennis	184	21 (11.4)	4 (2.2)
Triathlon	110	16 (14.5)	7 (6.4)
Volleyball	288	20 (6.9)	8 (2.8)
Weightlifting	252	44 (17.5)	10 (4.0)
Wrestling	343	41 (12.0)	16 (4.7)

Source: Adapted from Engebretsen *et al.* 2013. Reproduced with permission from BMJ Publishing Group Ltd.

Study design and population

The ability to describe the incidence, nature and causes of injuries and illnesses reliably has been recognised through the development of injury/illness surveillance consensus statements. Standardising

ABC of Sports and Exercise Medicine, Fourth Edition.
Edited by Gregory P. Whyte, Mike Loosemore and Clyde Williams.
© 2015 John Wiley & Sons, Ltd. Published 2015 by John Wiley & Sons, Ltd.

Table 1.2 Examples of injury and illness definitions used in epidemiological studies

a. Any physical complaint sustained by a player … irrespective of the need for medical-attention or time-loss from activities
b. Any musculoskeletal complaint … that received medical-attention regardless of the consequence with respect to absence from competition and/or training
c. Any physical complaint (not related to injury) that received medical-attention regardless of the consequence with respect to absence from competition and/or training
d. Any physical complaint sustained by a player during a match or training … that prevented the player from taking a full part in all … activities … for more than 1 day following the day of injury

study design and data collection makes it possible to compare results between studies. Firstly, the target population (or cohort) to be studied must be identified. Sometimes what defines a population is obvious, for example, in a study recording the number of injuries during the 2011 Rugby World Cup, the players competing during the World Cup are the population cohort. It is important to note the period of observation (i.e. again this may be naturally dictated by the cohort): who is going to record the data (i.e. team physician for medical data; coaches for training and competition exposure data), the methods of data collection (paper or electronic) and the type of study. Retrospective studies collect historical data over a set period of time, while prospective studies follow the cohort over a set future period of time. Prospective studies are generally more reliable than retrospective studies due to issues with the latter of memory recall bias, where even over short periods of time, more severe or more recent injuries and illness are likely to be remembered, but the less severe and more historical episodes are more likely to be forgotten.

Injury/illness definition

A universal definition of injury and illness, applicable to all sports, would be convenient and simple. Although this has not yet been achieved, the development of consensus statements has unified much of the research currently being undertaken (Table 1.2).

Classification of injuries and illnesses

The majority of epidemiological studies have focused on the aetiology of 'medical-attention' and/or 'time-loss' definitions of

injury and illness incidents, but few have related these events to an athlete's consequential physical limitations. For example, time-loss classifications are somewhat categorical in their use of the term (i.e. complete absence), when in reality many athletes continue to compete and train at high levels when experiencing pain and/or loss of function through injury or illness. Hence, there is a need to consider an additional level of classification focused on levels of impairment or performance restriction (Figure 1.1).

The classification and, therefore, the level of data collection required will need to be determined based on the study population, that is, recording all injuries including 'medical-attention' may not be appropriate for studies with large populations, or for contact sports (i.e. rugby) where the number of recorded injuries may be high, as this will create an overwhelming burden for recording on medical staff. Conversely, using a 'time-loss' only classification where there are a small number of acute traumatic injuries but an abundance of overuse chronic performance restriction injuries, for example, within swimming, may also not be appropriate. Once you have your injury and illness definition, it is this sub-classification that determines what becomes a recordable event. It is important to understand when comparing studies which injuries and illnesses are included, and which are excluded.

Rate of injury and illness

Reporting only absolute number of injuries or illnesses provides limited information about the risks to the sample population, without consideration for the volume or period of exposure to that risk, i.e., relative hours training/competing, number of athletes, number of weeks/months or seasons. The two most common methods of presenting the rate of injury or illness are incidence and prevalence. Traditionally, incidence is calculated taking the number of injuries (new and/or recurrent) divided by the total participant exposure time, and is presented as standard per 1000 h, to allow for inter-sport comparison. Incidence values for training and competition should always be reported separately (Table 1.3).

In the absence of hours of training and competition exposure, injuries can be expressed per 1000 athletes, or per 1000 athlete exposures (where one training session or competition run = 1 exposure). Unlike injuries, illnesses are not defined as occurring during training or competition hence are not usually expressed as a function of

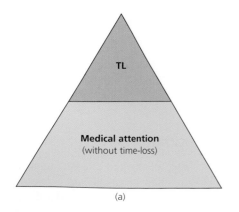

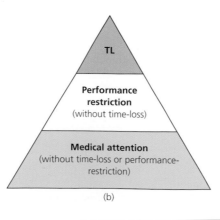

Figure 1.1 (a) Traditional hierarchy of injury/illness definition and classification, TL = time-loss.
(b) Alternative hierarchy of injury/illness definition and classification

Table 1.3 Example calculation for incidence of injury

A rugby club plays 48 matches in a season, during this time the players suffer 41 injuries

Exposure time	= 48 (matches) × 1.33 (length of match in hours)
	× 15 (number of players in the study team on pitch)
	= 960 player match hours
Incidence	= (41/960) × 1000
	= 43 injuries/1000 match hours

Table 1.4 Example calculation for prevalence of illness

A swimming squad of 45 athletes has 3 athletes suffer 4 illnesses during 1 week

Prevalence	= (3/45) × 100
	= 6.7%

Table 1.5 Example severity category grouping

Minimal	2–3 days
Mild	4–7 days
Moderate	8–28 days
Severe	>28 days

Table 1.6 Example risk factors for injury/illness

Risk factors	Examples
Time of season	Pre-season; month; week
Environment	Competition/match or training; playing position
Training	Sport specific; running; weight training; cardiovascular
Cause of injury	Contact; non-contact; acute traumatic; chronic overuse; recurrence
Location of injury	Head; shoulder; lumbar spine; thigh; knee; ankle
Type of injury	Sprain; fracture; concussion; contusion; tendinopathy
Affected illness system	Respiratory; gastrointestinal; cardiovascular; allergic; dental
Cause of illness	Infection; exercise induced; environmental; pre-existing

Table 1.7 Comparison of injury rate, severity and burden

Injury location	No. of injuries	Injury rate (%)	Average severity (days)	Total days lost	Burden (%)
Shoulder	3	6	17.6	52.8	7.5
Lumbar spine	5	12	24.5	122.5	17.5
Thigh	19	38	6.7	127.3	18.1
Knee	8	16	41.2	329.6	46.9
Ankle	14	28	5.0	70	10.0
Total	49	100	14.3	702.2	100

time (i.e. per 1000 athlete training or competition hours/exposures), but rather per 1000 athletes, or as prevalence.

Prevalence is used to calculate the proportion of the population that is injured or ill at a given time point (point prevalence) or over a set period of time (period prevalence). When calculating prevalence, it is important to remember that the number of individuals is key in expressing injury/illness as a percentage of the cohort (or team), rather than the absolute number of injuries or illnesses. For example, over the course of a season, a squad of 30 athletes may report 40 injuries, that is, multiple injuries per athlete. It is not possible to have more than 100% of the squad injured; hence, it is the number of athletes injured/ill out of the full squad of 30 that is calculated (Table 1.4).

Severity of injury and illness

The severity of injury and illness may be implicit in the level recorded, that is, an illness resulting in performance restriction versus complete time-loss, implies the latter illness is of greater severity. Traditionally, the number of days affected is the universally accepted way of reporting severity, and this is calculated as the number of days from the date of injury/illness to the date of return to full fitness. Days of severity may also be grouped within recommended severity categories (Table 1.5). In addition to the number of days, recording the level of pain on a visual analogue scale can provide an additional layer of information about the athletes' perception of the injury/illness severity.

Risk factors for injury and illness

Outcomes from epidemiological studies should include the rate and severity of injury and illness as a function of each risk factor, that is, location of injury and cause of illness (Table 1.6).

It is important to consider both what is most common and what is most severe when prioritising prevention strategies. For example, should efforts be focused on those injuries or illnesses that are most common (but maybe not very severe) or those that are most severe (but maybe not very common). An alternative way to answer this question would be to look at the total days lost or overall injury/illness burden (also known as risk), when determining overall importance for the direction of targeting prevention initiatives (Table 1.7).

Summary

Using sport injury/illness epidemiology consensus statements and common methodology will help produce valid and accurate study results, as well as allow inter-study comparisons to be made. The definition, rate and severity of injury and illness as well as more detailed information on the causes of injury/illness, relevant to the population of study, are key in correctly identifying areas of risk and allowing effective targeting of prevention initiatives.

Further reading

Brooks, J.H.M. & Fuller, C.W. (2006) The influence of methodological issues on the results and conclusions from epidemiological studies of sports injuries: illustrative examples. *Sports Medicine*, **36** (**6**), 459–472.

Engebretsen, L., Soligard, T., Steffen, K. *et al.* (2013) Sports injuries and illnesses during the London Summer Olympic Games 2012. *British Journal of Sports Medicine*, **47** (**7**), 407–414.

Fuller, C.W., Ekstrand, J., Junge, A. *et al.* (2006) Consensus statement on injury definitions and data collection procedures in studies of football (soccer) injuries. *British Journal of Sports Medicine*, **40** (**3**), 193–201.

Fuller, C.W., Sheerin, K. & Targett, S. (2013) Rugby World Cup 2011: International Rugby Board injury surveillance study. *British Journal of Sports Medicine*, **47**, 1184–1191.

van Mechelen, W., Hlobil, H. & Kemper, H. (1992) Incidence, severity, aetiology and prevention of sports injuries: a review of concepts. *Sports Medicine.*, **14**, 82–99.

Palmer-Green, D., Fuller, C., Jaques, R. *et al.* (2013) The Injury/Illness Performance Project (IIPP): a novel epidemiological approach for recording the consequences of sports injuries and illnesses. *Journal of Sports Medicine.* http://dx.doi.org/10.1155/2013/523974 [Article ID 523974, 9 pages]

CHAPTER 2

Immediate Care in Sport

Andy Smith

Mid Yorkshire Hospitals NHS Trust, Wakefield, England; Yorkshire Ambulance Service, Yorkshire, England; RFU Immediate Care in Sport Programme, Rugby Football Union, Twickenham, England; World Rugby Immediate Care in Rugby, World Rugby, Dublin, Ireland

---

> **OVERVIEW**
>
> After studying this chapter, the reader will understand the following:
> - Emergency action plan
> - Initial assessment and management
> - Spinal injury in sport
> - Musculoskeletal trauma
> - Wound care
> - Medical emergencies
> - Medical equipment

Introduction

Participation in sports at all levels is on the increase. Even though relatively rare, every year there are incidences in sport of significant trauma and/or medical emergencies.

At high exposure elite sporting events, there are often numerous medical personnel in attendance including doctors and paramedics to deliver immediate care if required. More often at non-elite events, there are limited personnel with adequate training and equipment to deal with the immediate care of the athletes.

> **Faculty of Pre Hospital Immediate Care in Sport Endorsed courses**
>
> - RFU immediate care in sport (ICIS)
> - SRU medical cardiac and pitch-side skills (SCRUMCAPS)
> - RFL immediate medical management on the field of play (IMMOF)
> - FA resuscitation and emergency aid (AREA)
> - IFSEM standard principles of resuscitation and trauma immediate care (SPoRTs)
> - Emergency medical management in individual and team sports (EMMiITS

There is a well-defined need for doctors, physiotherapists and other professionals looking after athletes and teams to be personally equipped with the skills and equipment required to deliver immediate care at the pitch side, race track, poolside and so on. It is the practitioners' duty that they are trained to the minimum level expected of their discipline and their skills are reviewed and refreshed regularly. These professionals do need to be prepared on not only match/event days but also at training venues and grounds where a significant number of injuries or medical problems can occur.

Emergency action planning

> **Emergency action plan**
>
> - Written emergency action plan that define roles minimises errors
> - Equipment maintenance and checks are essential
> - Risk assessment and plans inclusive of both training and match day venues
> - Establish minimum standards of medical equipment available at training venues, pitch side and travelling with athletes to away venue
> - Ensure knowledge of facilities at local hospitals and medical assistance/extrication team at the ground
> - Ensure medical team are aware of players and staff who have significant medical conditions

The quality of field of play care, effective team working and communication with the emergency services are crucial to a favourable outcome. Consideration to risk should be given to minimise factors that may impede effective immediate care and team working in the event of an emergency.

The development of an 'Emergency Action Plan' through a risk assessment that considers the sporting environment, communication, skill retention and team working in emergency situations is an essential part of immediate care preparedness in sport.

Such a plan should consider potential situations at both training and match venues and include standard operating procedures for particular scenarios as well as minimum standards of equipment and responsibilities with regard to equipment checking and skill maintenance of practitioners.

Initial assessment and management

The treatment of a seriously injured or ill player requires rapid initial assessment and initiation of the appropriate life- or limb-saving care

---

ABC of Sports and Exercise Medicine, Fourth Edition.
Edited by Gregory P. Whyte, Mike Loosemore and Clyde Williams.
© 2015 John Wiley & Sons, Ltd. Published 2015 by John Wiley & Sons, Ltd.

in a safe environment. Time is of the essence. A systematic approach is required to ensure injuries or the consequence of illness, are identified and treated in the correct order.

Systematic approach

- SAFE approach
- Primary survey with
- Resuscitation as required
- Re-evaluation
- Secondary survey
- Definitive care

SAFE approach

It is essential that the members of the medical team ensure that it is safe to approach the injured athlete. When entering the field of play, ensure your medical team know you are attending to an athlete and the officials are made aware. Wearing a brightly coloured bib may assist this.

SAFE approach

- Shout for help
- Assess the scene
- Free from danger
- Evaluate the player

Primary survey

Injured or critically ill athletes should be assessed and their treatment priorities should be established based on their mechanism of injury, injuries identified and vital signs. The vital signs must be assessed quickly and efficiently with management consisting of a rapid primary survey including resuscitation of identified problems and re-evaluation. This process constitutes of the <c>ABCDEs of immediate care. Life-threatening conditions should be identified and management should be commenced simultaneously.

Primary survey

- Catastrophic bleeding management
- Airway maintenance with C-spine protection
- Breathing with adequate ventilation
- Circulation with haemorrhage control
- Disability: neurological status
- Exposure and environment control

Catastrophic haemorrhage control

In the very rare circumstance of an athlete presenting with catastrophic haemorrhage, the application of a pressure dressing and the use of an arterial tourniquet or haemostatic agents should be considered in an attempt to arrest the bleeding before moving to assess and maintain the athlete's airway.

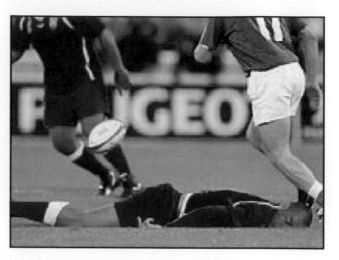

Figure 2.1 Unconscious player with unprotected airway

Airway maintenance with C-spine protection

In a suspected injured athlete if there is any possibility of a cervical spine injury, the neck must be controlled by manual in-line immobilisation as part of the initial approach (Figure 2.1). The airway assessment begins by assessing if the athlete is able to respond with a clear verbal response to voice commands. Listening to the quality of the voice may give information about the airway status and a clue to any impending problems.

It is essential to identify airway compromise early and manage this appropriately to minimise hypoxia and hypercarbia. Furthermore, it is important that the airway is regularly re-evaluated since some airway problems are progressive in nature and may not be apparent during the first primary survey.

Most episodes of airway obstruction can be easily managed with simple airway manoeuvres. The key to successful management is early recognition, and one must always be suspicious for actual or potential airway compromise. Situations necessitating more advanced interventions are rare in sport, but practitioners must be aware of the possibility of airway obstruction and be ready to manage it appropriately.

Breathing with adequate ventilation

It is important to determine the respiratory rate and to check for equal expansion of the chest wall. A cursory palpation of the chest wall at this time will reveal any areas of crepitus or tenderness. It is unlikely that an athlete will sustain an immediate life-threatening injury on the field of play, but if respiratory distress is identified a further assessment is required.

The more detailed assessment of breathing will normally take place in the medical room or ambulance where inspection of the thorax, respiratory rate, expansion, percussion and auscultation, and examination for tracheal deviation and cyanosis are undertaken.

Thankfully major chest trauma in sport is uncommon, but serious injuries do occur, and it is important that pitch-side care providers are able to diagnose and manage serious chest injuries. Life-threatening conditions should be identified, and appropriate immediate treatment delivered. All athletes with critical injury or illness should be provided with oxygen via a non-rebreath (trauma) mask with high-flow oxygen.

Circulation with haemorrhage control

Circulation assessment

- Pulse – presence of the radial pulse
- Pulse – rate and volume
- Colour of the player – noting pallor
- Mental status – conscious level and agitation
- Evidence of external bleeding
- Evidence of internal bleeding

It is essential through this systematic approach to recognise early signs of shock, and if haemorrhagic, attempt to stop or stem the bleeding while transferring the athlete to the appropriate emergency department for more definitive care.

The presence of the radial pulse usually indicates that the blood pressure is adequate for end-organ perfusion. It is used as a guide to whether intravenous fluids should be administered to an athlete in 250 ml aliquots of crystalloid, who has received blunt thoracic or abdominal trauma.

The presence of external haemorrhage should be managed by direct pressure to the wound and the application of dressings to stem the bleeding. If an athlete has clinical evidence of shock, it is important that all major areas of occult bleeding are assessed, namely the chest, abdomen, retroperitoneum, pelvis and long bones. Appropriate measures, for example, application of pelvic binder or immobilisation of long-bone fracture, should be undertaken if appropriate.

Disability: neurological status

The on-pitch baseline observation of the neurological status of the player involves the use of the AVPU system. Once, in the medical room, a more detailed neurological examination should be undertaken using the Glasgow Coma Scale (GCS). This should be repeated frequently and recorded along with all observations in the primary survey to identify improvement or deterioration in the player.

Field of play neurological assessment

- A – Alert
- V – Responding to voice
- P – Responding to painful stimulus
- U – Unresponsive

A significant head injury that occurs within the context of sport represents a medical emergency.

Efforts should be focused on meticulous cervical spine immobilisation at all times, early application of high-flow oxygen, attention to airway, breathing and circulation, safe extrication and transfer to the appropriate nearest emergency department if no improvement.

Any athlete suspected of having a concussion should be removed from play and assessed by a licensed healthcare provider trained in the evaluation and management of concussion. There is no perfect diagnostic test that clinicians can rely on; however, diagnosis involves the clinical assessment of a range of domains including symptoms, cognition and balance.

There is no same-day return to play for an athlete diagnosed with concussion. The mainstay of treatment is relative cognitive and physical rest until symptoms have resolved and then adherence to a graduated return to play protocol.

Exposure and environment control

For the initial field of play assessment, there should be limited exposure and the athlete protected from the environment. Once, in a more protected environment, the athlete may be exposed facilitating a thorough examination and assessment if time allows and does not delay transfer to definitive care.

Resuscitation

The management of life-threatening injuries/illness as they are identified is essential to optimise the athlete's condition. For example, airway problems must be treated immediately and corrected before assessment of breathing is commenced. All athletes who are suffering any significant illness or injury should have oxygen administered at 10–15 l/min via a well-fitting non-rebreath mask with an appropriately filled reservoir bag.

Re-evaluation

Re-evaluation of the player should be undertaken after any

- Intervention
- Deterioration
- Cause for concern
- Uncertainty

Continuous monitoring of vital signs and neurological status is essential. Athletes with significant injuries or illness must be re-evaluated constantly to ensure that new findings are not overlooked and to identify deterioration.

Secondary survey

An athlete with a time-critical illness or injury should never be detained in the pre-hospital setting in order to perform a secondary assessment if transport to the appropriate hospital is available.

The secondary survey includes history (SAMPLE) and a systematic head-to-toe examination designed to detect all of the athlete's injuries. Pre-prepared documentation including the athlete's personal details, contact details including a next of kin and the (AMP) parts of SAMPLE already completed, speeds up this process.

SAMPLE history

- S – Signs and symptoms
- A – Allergies
- M – Medications
- P – Past medical history
- L – Last meal and drink
- E – Events and environment of the injury/illness

Definitive care

Recorded observations and the SAMPLE history information should accompany the athlete to the hospital. Documentation of observations on copies of the local Emergency Department observation charts may assist in the continuity of care of the athlete.

The transport of critically injured or ill athletes should be undertaken by qualified ambulance crews with appropriate equipment immediately available in case of deterioration in the athlete's condition.

The mnemonic ATMIST has now been widely adopted by the ambulance service and pre-hospital care medical teams for the handover of trauma patients. This would be appropriate to be used for seriously injured athletes both when pre-alerting emergency departments and when giving a face-to-face handover.

ATMIST handover

- A – Age of the athlete (sex of athlete often also included)
- T – Time of the injury and expected time of arrival
- M – Mechanism of injury
- I – Injuries present and suspected
- S – Signs including physiological parameters
- T – Treatment given and needed

Spinal injury in sport

Indication of a spinal injury

- Suspicious mechanism of injury
- Reduction in conscious level
- Neurological signs or symptoms
- Distracting injury
- Midline cervical spine tenderness
- Intoxication with alcohol or drugs
- Unable to voluntary rotate neck >45°R and 45°L
- Unable to flex and extend

Although spinal cord injuries are rare in sport, they have a very high consequence and therefore it is important that those providing pitch-side care are able to recognise and manage spinal injuries appropriately (Figure 2.2). A high index of suspicion for a spinal injury should be considered. Removal from the field of play should be undertaken by an experienced and well-trained team having undertaken pre-event rehearsal of extrication procedures (Figure 2.3).

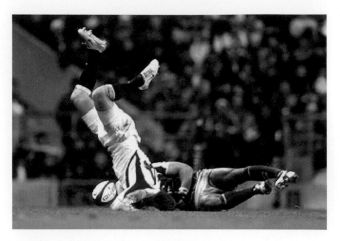

Figure 2.2 Suspicious mechanism for spinal injury

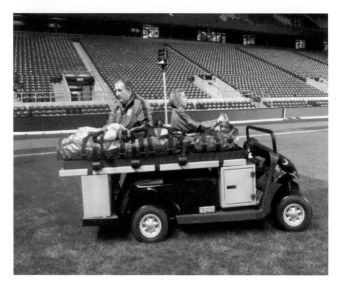

Figure 2.3 Safe extrication of a player with a suspected spinal injury

Musculoskeletal trauma

PRICE management of limb injuries

- Protect the injured limb from further injury
- Rest using a support or splint reduces movement and prevents further injury
- Ice provides direct pain relief and helps minimise swelling
- Compressing the injured muscle can provide support and prevent unnecessary movement
- Elevation if possible helps reduce swelling

Limb injuries are common in sport, and early appropriate management reduces the consequence of injury. Initial assessment should include assessing for open fractures, deformity and neurovascular compromise. Field-of-play management should include PRICE with effective analgesia, wound management, reduction and splinting achieving immobilisation of the injured limb.

Wound care

The correct management of sporting wounds is important if infection rates and other complications are to be kept to a minimum. All wounds sustained during sporting activities are dirty wounds. They require thorough cleaning, and exploration to assess and manage the full extent of any soft tissue damage before closure is undertaken. A temporising measure may be employed to allow quick return to play, but this must be removed after competition and the wound must be cleaned and treated appropriately. All wounds should be inspected regularly to check for signs of infection and treated appropriately.

Medical emergencies

There is a wide spectrum of medical conditions, including temperature-related illness that athletes and touring party members may have or succumb to. Some chronic medical conditions are relatively common among elite athletes, for example, asthma, allergies (anaphylaxis), diabetes and so on. Knowledge of such conditions is important, as is ensuring the medical team are aware of how to assess and manage these, with the correct medications and equipment.

The general approach to a player with a medical emergency is the same as one having sustained a traumatic injury: safe approach, ABCDE. As with any immediate care situation, definitive care with referral to a hospital emergency department should be considered early, and in any situation where a patient remains unstable, requires monitoring or is likely to relapse.

Medical equipment

Medical equipment should be maintained in accordance with the manufacturer's guidelines. A service log should be retained for all equipments and checklists recorded on at least a weekly basis. It is paramount that medical equipment is stored as directed by the manufacturer in secure and safe areas with appropriate security measures in place. The ordering, receiving, storage and disposal of medications including medical gases should be within the law.

Further reading

Faculty of Pre Hospital Care, Manual of Core Material (Royal College of Surgeons of Edinburgh)
Advanced Life Support Manual (Resuscitation Council UK)
Essential of Immediate Medical Care (C. John Eaton) (ISBN 0-443-05345-6)
Handbook of Immediate Medical Care (Greaves et al) (ISBN 0-7020-1881-3)
Practical Pre-hospital Care (Greaves et al) (ISBN 978-0-443-10360-5)
Pre-Hospital Care (Cooke) (ISBN 0-443-05987-X)
Pre-hospital Trauma Life Support Manual (ISBN 0-8151-6333-9)
Pre-Hospital Medicine (Greaves & Porter) (ISBN 0-340-67656-6)

CHAPTER 3

Head Injuries in Sport

Daniel G. Healy

Royal College of Surgeons, Ireland; National Neuroscience Centre, Beaumont hospital, Dublin, Ireland

---

OVERVIEW

- Concussion causes a variety of unrelated symptoms including headache, dizziness, mood disturbance, amnesia and foggy thinking.
- Linear and angular displacement causes a cascade of brain changes involving axonal, ion channel, inflammatory and mitochondrial dysfunction.
- Recurrent head injury significantly increases the risk of neurodegeneration in late middle age.
- Novel methods to visualise brain injury, measure the biochemical effects and predict risk will influence clinical practise in the future.

Introduction

Head injury is a common unwanted consequence of sport. In most cases, it is accidental. In combat sports such as boxing, it is intentional. Most head injuries are concussive and 80% resolve within 7–10 days. However, recovery time can be measured in months. Children/adolescents are more susceptible to concussion and prolonged recovery.

Serious head injury, for example, loss of consciousness or a clinical suspicion of haemorrhage, requires immediate brain scanning. This also applies where there is clinical uncertainty about the severity of the head injury.

Validated protocol-driven strategies are increasingly used in (i) the pre-assessment of athletes, for example, establishing baseline pre-season cognitive function and (ii) sideline management, for example, removal of ALL suspected concussed athletes from play. In general, these protocols are based on consensus expert opinion rather than scientific study.

Chronic traumatic encephalopathy (CTE) is a progressive incurable neurodegenerative disorder resulting in premature parkinsonism and dementia. CTE is unique to individuals exposed to recurrent head injury.

Epidemiology of head injury in sport

One in five head injuries in young adults are directly attributable to sport and recreation. It is difficult to make direct risk comparisons between sports. For example, in 2009, cycling accounted for the greatest number of head injuries (86,000 of 447,000 sports-related hospital head injuries in United States), followed by American football (47,000) yet cycling is clearly safer when directly compared with a sport like mixed-martial-arts (MMA); one-third of professional MMA contests results in an unconscious fighter or a technical knockout by head trauma.

Clear differences in concussion risk between male and female athletes have not been demonstrated for many sports; however, in some sports with identical male–female rules (basketball and soccer) concussion risk appears to be higher for female athletes. Rates are also higher in competition than during practice. Not all brain injury involves head trauma; for example, body-checking in ice hockey and rugby tackles also induce brain acceleration–deceleration injury. Furthermore, many concussions go unreported.

Types of head injury

Head injury can be separated into (i) concussion and (ii) those associated with demonstrable abnormality on brain scans, that is, neurosurgical-type head injury.

Concussion

The American Academy of Neurology defines concussion as a clinical syndrome of biomechanically induced alteration of brain function, typically affecting memory and orientation, which may involve loss of consciousness. This unwieldy definition underpins difficulty in defining a collection of self-reported symptoms with few objective clinical signs. Etymologically, the term concussion derives from the Latin verb concutere (to shake violently), which biomechanically depicts the brain injury. Ambroise Paré, a 16th-century military surgeon, succinctly used the subjective term – commotio cerebri (commotion of the brain) – a term still occasionally used.

Almost nothing is known about minor or 'sub-concussive' head injury except that most field-sport athletes sustain hundreds per season.

Symptoms and signs of concussion

The symptoms of concussion accord with the neuroanatomy. Injury to the mesial temporal lobes causes amnesia, frontal lobes/amygdala causes behavioural change/emotionality, and disruption to monoamine pathways of the brainstem, hypothalamus and basal forebrain causes insomnia.

It can be helpful to consider concussive symptoms as three categories:

1 **Somatic** (physical), for example, headache, unsteadiness, nausea, dizziness
2 **Cognitive**, for example, amnesia, slow reaction times, fogginess
3 **Behavioural**, for example, insomnia, irritability, emotional lability, drug abuse

Somatic symptoms tend to predominate acutely, whereas the cognitive-behavioural symptoms may not become apparent for hours to days when the effects of adrenaline have worn off. These symptoms are summarised in the Symptom Evaluation section of the Sports Concussion Assessment Tool (SCAT3) developed in Zurich by expert consensus (Figure 3.1). This document can be downloaded without copyright infringement (http://bjsm.bmj .com/content/47/5/259.full.pdf). A children's version is available. The pocket Concussion Recognition Tool is practical for pitchside assessments (http://bjsm.bmj.com/content/47/5/267.full.pdf).

A number of clinical points are worth considering.

Firstly, up to half of all concussions have delayed or unclear timing of symptom onset. Sometimes the association with antecedent head trauma is overlooked. Another common error is to downplay concussion because of the absence of loss of conscious that correlates more with the neuroanatomy of the injury rather than with actual injury severity. When loss of consciousness does occur, there is often a stereotypical recovery sequence that was richly described in 1932 by Ritchie Russell (Box 3.1).

Post-concussion headache frequently has migraineous qualities (e.g. nausea, photophobia, worsened by movement). Migraineurs *per se* may be more susceptible to concussion. Benign exercise-induced migraine is occasionally confused with concussion, and specialist neurological input is advised. It is also important to distinguish post-concussion headache from secondary causes needing neurosurgery (see later). Similarly, neck pain, common in concussion, can be confused with spinal injury.

Athletes use the term 'dizziness' interchangeably to describe a myriad of aetiologically unrelated symptoms: unsteadiness (cerebellum), vertigo (labyrinth) and impaired depth perception (parieto-occipital cortex). Most 'dizzy' symptoms predict slower than normal recovery. Concussive dizziness should be distinguished from true labyrinthine vertigo where the athlete's world spins violently around them invariably associated with objective signs of nystagmus. The most common cause in sport is benign positional paroxysmal vertigo (BPPV) where tiny dislodged otoconia (ear stones) stimulate the semicircular canals. Sudden head-turns provoke intense short-lasting (5–15 s) vertigo and severe rotatory nystagmus. BPPV is effectively cured by Epley's vestibular rehabilitation manoeuvres. In choking sports such as wrestling and MMA, 'dizziness' with neck pain raises the possibility of vertebral artery dissection and brainstem stroke.

Psychological symptoms may be the sole manifestation of concussion in adolescents. Uncharacteristic behavioural change, irritability, anger outbursts and drug abuse are red flags.

Finally, brief tonic posturing of the head or arm immediate to head impact is well recognised. Sometimes a 'fencing posture' is adopted, and there are rewarding examples searching this term in YouTube. Brief myoclonic jerks and concussive seizures are other phenomena seen. Although these indicate significant head injury, they do not confer an increase risk of epilepsy. In most countries, concussive seizures do not preclude driving and anti-epileptic medication is not needed.

Pathophysiology of concussion

The soft jelly-like brain can undergo linear acceleration–deceleration and/or angular (rotational) injury (Figure 3.2). Linear impact occurs when the accelerating head is suddenly stopped, and the free moving brain impacts the anterior inner hard skull bone. The resulting 'coup' injury may damage neurones at the site of impact while secondary rebound displacement or bouncing may impact the brain at sites opposite to the original impact (contra-coup). Direct blows to the occiput can mechanically elicit crude visual cortex activation explaining the 'seeing stars' phenomenon.

In angular acceleration, for example, a left hook punch to the jaw, the cortex twists upon the relatively fixed brainstem beneath it. This stretches axons causing the temporary dysfunction of upper brainstem centres important for consciousness (reticular activating centre) and limb tone (reticulospinal tracts). This explains the propensity of angular acceleration impacts to cause sudden loss of consciousness (flash KO) and/or transient limb hypotonia (jelly legs). In severe angular acceleration, for example, motor-racing crashes, the twisting process may shear axons resulting in severe cognitive and motor deficits. This 'diffuse axonal injury' affects white matter tracts such as the corpus callosum and inputs to the cerebellum. Diffusion tensor MRI imaging is increasingly used in clinical practice to measure this.

Head injury research in mice shows that trauma induces microscopic holes in the meninges and glial limitans sequentially followed

---

Box 3.1 **These classic lines penned in 1932 by Ritchie Russell describe the recovery sequence after a sporting head injury**

The first attempt to articulate usually takes the form of a groan or a shout repeated frequently. Then a few words are occasionally uttered. These may be meaningless, but soon a few common phrases are correctly produced. These are often repeated frequently and are usually shouted out loudly. The patient's vocabulary gradually increases. Common phrases are at first all that can be said, but gradually speech becomes more intelligible. There is still, however, a lack of any power of understanding or reason. The patient's incessant talk is mainly repetition. He pays no attention to what is said to him and is quite disorientated. The inhibitions and social training which prompt the average patient to speak with respect to the nurses and doctor are among the last functions to recover, so that he is often impudent to and familiar with his attendants. Subsequent to this stage the recovery of insight, orientation and the usual social habits rapidly follows, and the patient recovers full consciousness and begins to think about events preceding his accident.

Source: Russell, "Cerebral involvement in head injury"

SCAT3™

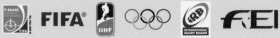

Sport Concussion Assessment Tool – 3rd Edition

For use by medical professionals only

Name	Date/Time of Injury:	Examiner:
	Date of Assessment:	

What is the SCAT3?[1]

The SCAT3 is a standardized tool for evaluating injured athletes for concussion and can be used in athletes aged from 13 years and older. It supersedes the original SCAT and the SCAT2 published in 2005 and 2009, respectively[2]. For younger persons, ages 12 and under, please use the Child SCAT3. The SCAT3 is designed for use by medical professionals. If you are not qualified, please use the Sport Concussion Recognition Tool[1]. Preseason baseline testing with the SCAT3 can be helpful for interpreting post-injury test scores.

Specific instructions for use of the SCAT3 are provided on page 3. If you are not familiar with the SCAT3, please read through these instructions carefully. This tool may be freely copied in its current form for distribution to individuals, teams, groups and organizations. Any revision or any reproduction in a digital form requires approval by the Concussion in Sport Group.
NOTE: The diagnosis of a concussion is a clinical judgment, ideally made by a medical professional. The SCAT3 should not be used solely to make, or exclude, the diagnosis of concussion in the absence of clinical judgement. An athlete may have a concussion even if their SCAT3 is "normal".

What is a concussion?

A concussion is a disturbance in brain function caused by a direct or indirect force to the head. It results in a variety of non-specific signs and/or symptoms (some examples listed below) and most often does not involve loss of consciousness. Concussion should be suspected in the presence of **any one or more** of the following:

- Symptoms (e.g., headache), or
- Physical signs (e.g., unsteadiness), or
- Impaired brain function (e.g. confusion) or
- Abnormal behaviour (e.g., change in personality).

SIDELINE ASSESSMENT

Indications for Emergency Management

NOTE: A hit to the head can sometimes be associated with a more serious brain injury. Any of the following warrants consideration of activating emergency procedures and urgent transportation to the nearest hospital:

- Glasgow Coma score less than 15
- Deteriorating mental status
- Potential spinal injury
- Progressive, worsening symptoms or new neurologic signs

Potential signs of concussion?

If any of the following signs are observed after a direct or indirect blow to the head, the athlete should stop participation, be evaluated by a medical professional and **should not be permitted to return to sport the same day** if a concussion is suspected.

Any loss of consciousness?	Y	N
"If so, how long?" _____		
Balance or motor incoordination (stumbles, slow/laboured movements, etc.)?	Y	N
Disorientation or confusion (inability to respond appropriately to questions)?	Y	N
Loss of memory:	Y	N
"If so, how long?" _____		
"Before or after the injury?" _____		
Blank or vacant look:	Y	N
Visible facial injury in combination with any of the above:	Y	N

1 Glasgow coma scale (GCS)

Best eye response (E)

No eye opening	1
Eye opening in response to pain	2
Eye opening to speech	3
Eyes opening spontaneously	4

Best verbal response (V)

No verbal response	1
Incomprehensible sounds	2
Inappropriate words	3
Confused	4
Oriented	5

Best motor response (M)

No motor response	1
Extension to pain	2
Abnormal flexion to pain	3
Flexion/Withdrawal to pain	4
Localizes to pain	5
Obeys commands	6

Glasgow Coma score (E + V + M)	of 15

GCS should be recorded for all athletes in case of subsequent deterioration.

2 Maddocks Score[3]

"I am going to ask you a few questions, please listen carefully and give your best effort."
Modified Maddocks questions (1 point for each correct answer)

What venue are we at today?	0	1
Which half is it now?	0	1
Who scored last in this match?	0	1
What team did you play last week/game?	0	1
Did your team win the last game?	0	1
Maddocks score		of 5

Maddocks score is validated for sideline diagnosis of concussion only and is not used for serial testing.

Notes: Mechanism of Injury (**"tell me what happened"**?):

_____

_____

_____

_____

Any athlete with a suspected concussion should be REMOVED FROM PLAY, medically assessed, monitored for deterioration (i.e., should not be left alone) and should not drive a motor vehicle until cleared to do so by a medical professional. No athlete diagnosed with concussion should be returned to sports participation on the day of Injury.

Figure 3.1 The Sports Concussion Assessment Tool (SCAT3) developed in Zurich by expert consensus for evaluating concussion and can be used in athletes older than 13 years. SCAT3 is a screening evaluation tool and does not independently determine the diagnosis of a concussion or return to play status. Such determination can only be made by a medical professional with experience in the treatment of concussion. © 2013 Concussion in Sport Group

BACKGROUND

Name: _____ Date: _____

Examiner: _____

Sport/team/school: _____ Date/time of injury: _____

Age: _____ Gender: ☐ M ☐ F

Years of education completed: _____

Dominant hand: ☐ right ☐ left ☐ neither

How many concussions do you think you have had in the past? _____

When was the most recent concussion? _____

How long was your recovery from the most recent concussion? _____

Have you ever been hospitalized or had medical imaging done for a head injury? ☐ Y ☐ N

Have you ever been diagnosed with headaches or migraines? ☐ Y ☐ N

Do you have a learning disability, dyslexia, ADD/ADHD? ☐ Y ☐ N

Have you ever been diagnosed with depression, anxiety or other psychiatric disorder? ☐ Y ☐ N

Has anyone in your family ever been diagnosed with any of these problems? ☐ Y ☐ N

Are you on any medications? If yes, please list: ☐ Y ☐ N

SCAT3 to be done in resting state. Best done 10 or more minutes post excercise.

SYMPTOM EVALUATION

3 How do you feel?

"You should score yourself on the following symptoms, based on how you feel now".

	none	mild		moderate		severe	
Headache	0	1	2	3	4	5	6
"Pressure in head"	0	1	2	3	4	5	6
Neck Pain	0	1	2	3	4	5	6
Nausea or vomiting	0	1	2	3	4	5	6
Dizziness	0	1	2	3	4	5	6
Blurred vision	0	1	2	3	4	5	6
Balance problems	0	1	2	3	4	5	6
Sensitivity to light	0	1	2	3	4	5	6
Sensitivity to noise	0	1	2	3	4	5	6
Feeling slowed down	0	1	2	3	4	5	6
Feeling like "in a fog"	0	1	2	3	4	5	6
"Don't feel right"	0	1	2	3	4	5	6
Difficulty concentrating	0	1	2	3	4	5	6
Difficulty remembering	0	1	2	3	4	5	6
Fatigue or low energy	0	1	2	3	4	5	6
Confusion	0	1	2	3	4	5	6
Drowsiness	0	1	2	3	4	5	6
Trouble falling asleep	0	1	2	3	4	5	6
More emotional	0	1	2	3	4	5	6
Irritability	0	1	2	3	4	5	6
Sadness	0	1	2	3	4	5	6
Nervous or Anxious	0	1	2	3	4	5	6

Total number of symptoms (Maximum possible 22) ☐

Symptom severity score (Maximum possible 132) ☐

Do the symptoms get worse with physical activity? ☐ Y ☐ N

Do the symptoms get worse with mental activity? ☐ Y ☐ N

☐ self rated ☐ self rated and clinician monitored

☐ clinician interview ☐ self rated with parent input

Overall rating: If you know the athlete well prior to the injury, how different is the athlete acting compared to his/her usual self?

Please circle one response:

no different	very different	unsure	N/A

Scoring on the SCAT3 should not be used as a stand-alone method to diagnose concussion, measure recovery or make decisions about an athlete's readiness to return to competition after concussion. Since signs and symptoms may evolve over time, it is important to consider repeat evaluation in the acute assessment of concussion.

COGNITIVE & PHYSICAL EVALUATION

4 Cognitive assessment
Standardized Assessment of Concussion (SAC)[4]

Orientation (1 point for each correct answer)

What month is it?	0	1
What is the date today?	0	1
What is the day of the week?	0	1
What year is it?	0	1
What time is it right now? (within 1 hour)	0	1
Orientation score		of 5

Immediate memory

List	Trial 1		Trial 2		Trial 3		Alternative word list		
elbow	0	1	0	1	0	1	candle	baby	finger
apple	0	1	0	1	0	1	paper	monkey	penny
carpet	0	1	0	1	0	1	sugar	perfume	blanket
saddle	0	1	0	1	0	1	sandwich	sunset	lemon
bubble	0	1	0	1	0	1	wagon	iron	insect
Total									

Immediate memory score total   of 15

Concentration: Digits Backward

List	Trial 1		Alternative digit list		
4-9-3	0	1	6-2-9	5-2-6	4-1-5
3-8-1-4	0	1	3-2-7-9	1-7-9-5	4-9-6-8
6-2-9-7-1	0	1	1-5-2-8-6	3-8-5-2-7	6-1-8-4-3
7-1-8-4-6-2	0	1	5-3-9-1-4-8	8-3-1-9-6-4	7-2-4-8-5-6
Total of 4					

Concentration: Month in Reverse Order (1 pt. for entire sequence correct)

Dec-Nov-Oct-Sept-Aug-Jul-Jun-May-Apr-Mar-Feb-Jan   0   1

Concentration score   of 5

5 Neck Examination:

Range of motion   Tenderness   Upper and lower limb sensation & strength

Findings:

6 Balance examination

Do one or both of the following tests.

Footwear (shoes, barefoot, braces, tape, etc.) _____

Modified Balance Error Scoring System (BESS) testing[5]

Which foot was tested (i.e. which is the non-dominant foot) ☐ Left ☐ Right

Testing surface (hard floor, field, etc.) _____

Condition

Double leg stance:	Errors
Single leg stance (non-dominant foot):	Errors
Tandem stance (non-dominant foot at back):	Errors

And/Or

Tandem gait[6,7]

Time (best of 4 trials): _____ seconds

7 Coordination examination
Upper limb coordination

Which arm was tested: ☐ Left ☐ Right

Coordination score   of 1

8 SAC Delayed Recall[4]

Delayed recall score   of 5

Figure 3.1 *(continued)*

INSTRUCTIONS

Words in *Italics* throughout the SCAT3 are the instructions given to the athlete by the tester.

Symptom Scale

"You should score yourself on the following symptoms, based on how you feel now".

To be completed by the athlete. In situations where the symptom scale is being completed after exercise, it should still be done in a resting state, at least 10 minutes post exercise.

For total number of symptoms, maximum possible is 22.

For Symptom severity score, add all scores in table, maximum possible is 22 x 6 = 132.

SAC[4]

Immediate Memory

"I am going to test your memory. I will read you a list of words and when I am done, repeat back as many words as you can remember, in any order."

Trials 2 & 3:

"I am going to repeat the same list again. Repeat back as many words as you can remember in any order, even if you said the word before."

Complete all 3 trials regardless of score on trial 1 & 2. Read the words at a rate of one per second. **Score 1 pt. for each correct response.** Total score equals sum across all 3 trials. Do not inform the athlete that delayed recall will be tested.

Concentration

Digits backward

"I am going to read you a string of numbers and when I am done, you repeat them back to me backwards, in reverse order of how I read them to you. For example, if I say 7-1-9, you would say 9-1-7."

If correct, go to next string length. If incorrect, read trial 2. **One point possible for each string length.** Stop after incorrect on both trials. The digits should be read at the rate of one per second.

Months in reverse order

"Now tell me the months of the year in reverse order. Start with the last month and go backward. So you'll say December, November … Go ahead"

1 pt. for entire sequence correct

Delayed Recall

The delayed recall should be performed after completion of the Balance and Coordination Examination.

"Do you remember that list of words I read a few times earlier? Tell me as many words from the list as you can remember in any order."

Score 1 pt. for each correct response

Balance Examination

Modified Balance Error Scoring System (BESS) testing[5]

This balance testing is based on a modified version of the Balance Error Scoring System (BESS)[5]. A stopwatch or watch with a second hand is required for this testing.

"I am now going to test your balance. Please take your shoes off, roll up your pant legs above ankle (if applicable), and remove any ankle taping (if applicable). This test will consist of three twenty second tests with different stances."

(a) Double leg stance:

"The first stance is standing with your feet together with your hands on your hips and with your eyes closed. You should try to maintain stability in that position for 20 seconds. I will be counting the number of times you move out of this position. I will start timing when you are set and have closed your eyes."

(b) Single leg stance:

"If you were to kick a ball, which foot would you use? [This will be the dominant foot] Now stand on your non-dominant foot. The dominant leg should be held in approximately 30 degrees of hip flexion and 45 degrees of knee flexion. Again, you should try to maintain stability for 20 seconds with your hands on your hips and your eyes closed. I will be counting the number of times you move out of this position. If you stumble out of this position, open your eyes and return to the start position and continue balancing. I will start timing when you are set and have closed your eyes."

(c) Tandem stance:

"Now stand heel-to-toe with your non-dominant foot in back. Your weight should be evenly distributed across both feet. Again, you should try to maintain stability for 20 seconds with your hands on your hips and your eyes closed. I will be counting the number of times you move out of this position. If you stumble out of this position, open your eyes and return to the start position and continue balancing. I will start timing when you are set and have closed your eyes."

Balance testing – types of errors

1. Hands lifted off iliac crest
2. Opening eyes
3. Step, stumble, or fall
4. Moving hip into > 30 degrees abduction
5. Lifting forefoot or heel
6. Remaining out of test position > 5 sec

Each of the 20-second trials is scored by counting the errors, or deviations from the proper stance, accumulated by the athlete. The examiner will begin counting errors only after the individual has assumed the proper start position. **The modified BESS is calculated by adding one error point for each error during the three 20-second tests. The maximum total number of errors for any single condition is 10.** If an athlete commits multiple errors simultaneously, only one error is recorded but the athlete should quickly return to the testing position, and counting should resume once subject is set. Subjects that are unable to maintain the testing procedure for a minimum of **five seconds** at the start are assigned the highest possible score, ten, for that testing condition.

OPTION: For further assessment, the same 3 stances can be performed on a surface of medium density foam (e.g., approximately 50 cm x 40 cm x 6 cm).

Tandem Gait[6,7]

Participants are instructed to stand with their feet together behind a starting line (the test is best done with footwear removed). Then, they walk in a forward direction as quickly and as accurately as possible along a 38mm wide (sports tape), 3 meter line with an alternate foot heel-to-toe gait ensuring that they approximate their heel and toe on each step. Once they cross the end of the 3m line, they turn 180 degrees and return to the starting point using the same gait. A total of 4 trials are done and the best time is retained. Athletes should complete the test in 14 seconds. Athletes fail the test if they step off the line, have a separation between their heel and toe, or if they touch or grab the examiner or an object. In this case, the time is not recorded and the trial repeated, if appropriate.

Coordination Examination

Upper limb coordination

Finger-to-nose (FTN) task:

"I am going to test your coordination now. Please sit comfortably on the chair with your eyes open and your arm (either right or left) outstretched (shoulder flexed to 90 degrees and elbow and fingers extended), pointing in front of you. When I give a start signal, I would like you to perform five successive finger to nose repetitions using your index finger to touch the tip of the nose, and then return to the starting position, as quickly and as accurately as possible."

Scoring: 5 correct repetitions in < 4 seconds = 1
Note for testers: Athletes fail the test if they do not touch their nose, do not fully extend their elbow or do not perform five repetitions. **Failure should be scored as 0.**

References & Footnotes

1. This tool has been developed by a group of international experts at the 4th International Consensus meeting on Concussion in Sport held in Zurich, Switzerland in November 2012. The full details of the conference outcomes and the authors of the tool are published in The BJSM Injury Prevention and Health Protection, 2013, Volume 47, Issue 5. The outcome paper will also be simultaneously co-published in other leading biomedical journals with the copyright held by the Concussion in Sport Group, to allow unrestricted distribution, providing no alterations are made.

2. McCrory P et al., Consensus Statement on Concussion in Sport – the 3rd International Conference on Concussion in Sport held in Zurich, November 2008. British Journal of Sports Medicine 2009; 43: i76-89.

3. Maddocks, DL; Dicker, GD; Saling, MM. The assessment of orientation following concussion in athletes. Clinical Journal of Sport Medicine. 1995; 5(1): 32–3.

4. McCrea M. Standardized mental status testing of acute concussion. Clinical Journal of Sport Medicine. 2001; 11: 176–181.

5. Guskiewicz KM. Assessment of postural stability following sport-related concussion. Current Sports Medicine Reports. 2003; 2: 24–30.

6. Schneiders, A.G., Sullivan, S.J., Gray, A., Hammond-Tooke, G. & McCrory, P. Normative values for 16-37 year old subjects for three clinical measures of motor performance used in the assessment of sports concussions. Journal of Science and Medicine in Sport. 2010; 13(2): 196–201.

7. Schneiders, A.G., Sullivan, S.J., Kvarnstrom. J.K., Olsson, M., Yden. T. & Marshall, S.W. The effect of footwear and sports-surface on dynamic neurological screening in sport-related concussion. Journal of Science and Medicine in Sport. 2010; 13(4): 382–386

Figure 3.1 *(continued)*

ATHLETE INFORMATION

Any athlete suspected of having a concussion should be removed from play, and then seek medical evaluation.

Signs to watch for

Problems could arise over the first 24–48 hours. The athlete should not be left alone and must go to a hospital at once if they:

- Have a headache that gets worse
- Are very drowsy or can't be awakened
- Can't recognize people or places
- Have repeated vomiting
- Behave unusually or seem confused; are very irritable
- Have seizures (arms and legs jerk uncontrollably)
- Have weak or numb arms or legs
- Are unsteady on their feet; have slurred speech

Remember, it is better to be safe.
Consult your doctor after a suspected concussion.

Return to play

Athletes should not be returned to play the same day of injury.
When returning athletes to play, they should be **medically cleared and then follow a stepwise supervised program,** with stages of progression.

For example:

Rehabilitation stage	Functional exercise at each stage of rehabilitation	Objective of each stage
No activity	Physical and cognitive rest	Recovery
Light aerobic exercise	Walking, swimming or stationary cycling keeping intensity, 70% maximum predicted heart rate. No resistance training	Increase heart rate
Sport-specific exercise	Skating drills in ice hockey, running drills in soccer. No head impact activities	Add movement
Non-contact training drills	Progression to more complex training drills, eg passing drills in football and ice hockey. May start progressive resistance training	Exercise, coordination, and cognitive load
Full contact practice	Following medical clearance participate in normal training activities	Restore confidence and assess functional skills by coaching staff
Return to play	Normal game play	

There should be at least 24 hours (or longer) for each stage and if symptoms recur the athlete should rest until they resolve once again and then resume the program at the previous asymptomatic stage. Resistance training should only be added in the later stages.

If the athlete is symptomatic for more than 10 days, then consultation by a medical practitioner who is expert in the management of concussion, is recommended.

Medical clearance should be given before return to play.

Scoring Summary:

Test Domain	Score		
	Date: _____	Date: _____	Date: _____
Number of Symptoms of 22			
Symptom Severity Score of 132			
Orientation of 5			
Immediate Memory of 15			
Concentration of 5			
Delayed Recall of 5			
SAC Total			
BESS (total errors)			
Tandem Gait (seconds)			
Coordination of 1			

Notes:

_____
_____
_____
_____
_____
_____
_____
_____
_____
_____
_____
_____
_____
_____
_____
_____

✂ -

CONCUSSION INJURY ADVICE

(To be given to the **person monitoring** the concussed athlete)

This patient has received an injury to the head. A careful medical examination has been carried out and no sign of any serious complications has been found. Recovery time is variable across individuals and the patient will need monitoring for a further period by a responsible adult. Your treating physician will provide guidance as to this timeframe.

If you notice any change in behaviour, vomiting, dizziness, worsening headache, double vision or excessive drowsiness, please contact your doctor or the nearest hospital emergency department immediately.

Other important points:

- Rest (physically and mentally), including training or playing sports until symptoms resolve and you are medically cleared
- No alcohol
- No prescription or non-prescription drugs without medical supervision. Specifically:
  · No sleeping tablets
  · Do not use aspirin, anti-inflammatory medication or sedating pain killers
- Do not drive until medically cleared
- Do not train or play sport until medically cleared

Clinic phone number

Patient's name _____

Date/time of injury _____

Date/time of medical review _____

Treating physician _____

Contact details or stamp

Figure 3.1 (continued)

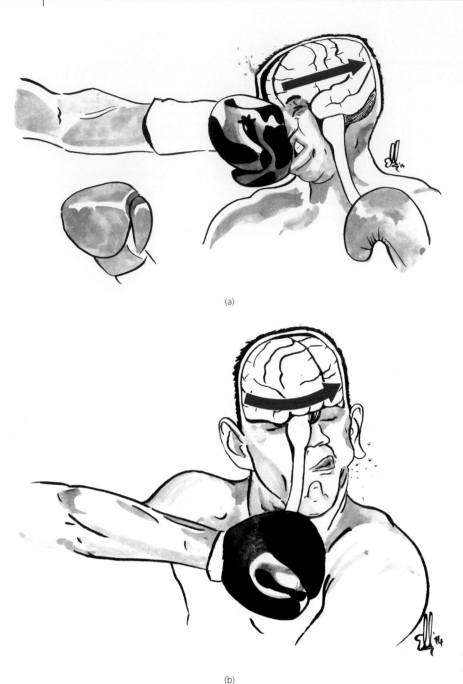

(a)

(b)

Figure 3.2 Schematic depiction of head trauma causing linear acceleration–deceleration (a) and angular brain rotation (b). Drawings made by Dr Eoin Kelleher (www.eoinkelleher.com)

by neuronal loss. The brain's inflammatory responses, in particular microglia, plug these holes implying that inflammation in mild traumatic brain injury may be beneficial. Meningeal signal change may be seen in up to 50% of concussed athletes using FLAIR T2 sequences on standard MRI machines.

At a single-cell level, a cascade of metabolic processes occurs initiated by an indiscriminate release of neurotransmitters such as glutamate. This alters ion-channel flux causing the extracellular egress of potassium ions and intracellular movement of calcium. The energy (ATP/glucose) required for restoring normal ion gradients may trigger a cellular energy crisis. Reduced Positron Emission Tomoraphy (PET) scan glucose uptake is seen in the injured brain regions of concussed athletes.

In CSF, abnormally high levels of important brain proteins (tau, neurofilament, S100B) are seen. The antibodies to astrocytic protein S100B have been found in the serum of American football players, raising the possibility of blood–brain barrier injury and a pathogenic immune response. The measurement of such biomarker proteins may play an important role in the diagnosis of concussion. Moreover, in the future, it may be that players can only return-to-play after the energy deficits on PET brain scans or the protein rises in blood and CSF have normalised.

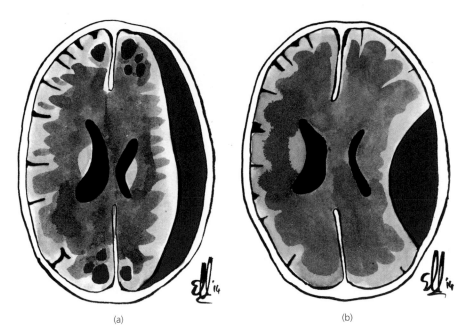

(a)　　　　　　　　(b)

Figure 3.3 Schematic representation of subdural brain haemorrhage of the left temporal lobe and the associated coup and contra-coup intraparenchymal haemorrhage or contusion (a) and extradural brain haemorrhage of left temporal lobe (b). Drawings made by Dr Eoin Kelleher (www.eoinkelleher.com)

Neurosurgical head injury

Serious head trauma may lead to intracranial haemorrhage involving either brain parenchyma or the surrounding subdural or extradural meningeal spaces (Figure 3.3). Subdural bleeding tends to be venous (bridging veins), and therefore symptoms progress more slowly than the typically arterial bleeding of extradural haemorrhage (often associated with skull fracture and rupture of the middle meningeal artery).

Clinical signs of neurosurgical head injury include peri-orbital and post-auricular ecchymosis (Battle's sign), haemotympanum, CSF otorrhoea/rhinorrhoea and facial fractures. Careful evaluation for optic nerve swelling (papilloedema) is an imperative as it is an important clue to raised intracranial pressure.

There is considerable overlap between the symptoms of neurosurgical head injury and concussion. Severe headache, post-traumatic amnesia, age greater than 65 years, seizures (5–10%) and focal neurological deficits (e.g. pupil asymmetry from midbrain compression) are red flags. The definitive tests are CT and MRI brain scans. MRI offers a more rigorous evaluation of brain parenchyma especially for small haemorrhage. However, early haemorrhage is easier seen on CT.

The main risk of haemorrhage (and associated oedema) is transtentorial temporal lobe herniation and the compression of brainstem or vascular structures (coning). Haematoma evacuation and intracranial pressure monitoring are required in such cases. Small haematomas, not associated with significant intracranial pressure, are usually managed conservatively. A caveat of extradural haemorrhage is that 30% of athletes have a 'the lucid interval'; an athlete is knocked unconscious by initial concussive forces but recovers quickly (lucid interval) only to relapse unconscious minutes to hours later when unrecognised extradural bleeding causes secondary raised intracranial pressure. This is one reason why all head injury athletes should be observed for at least 24 h (including waking from sleep) and alcohol avoided.

Long-term post-traumatic psychological changes to mood, motivation and personality are common after intraparenchymal frontal lobe trauma. Approximately 10% of athletes develop unprovoked epileptic seizures within 5 years.

Second impact syndrome

This is where the brain undergoes diffuse uncontrolled swelling after a second, often minor, impact. Transtentorial herniation ensues. The mechanism is unclear but loss of the autoregulation of cerebral blood flow is cited. Calcium channel dysregulation may be another explanation.

Second impact syndrome is rare and more common in children/adolescents. Some cases may simply be late effects of the first impact.

Head injury management

Serious brain injury impairs the respiratory patterns in the unconscious/semiconscious athlete. Immediate management should incorporate Advanced Trauma Life Support (ATLS) guidelines. A rapid primary survey should be performed using the core 'ABCDE' principles. Appropriate airway management may prevent and limit secondary hypoxic brain injury.

The placement of a definitive airway is the gold standard of airway care. This usually requires the use of an induction agent and a short-acting neuromuscular blocking agent by personnel experienced in advanced airway care. However, this expertise and equipment is rarely available at sporting events. An exception to this is professional boxing where an anaesthetist is usually ringside. The physical environment of the incident may hamper resuscitation

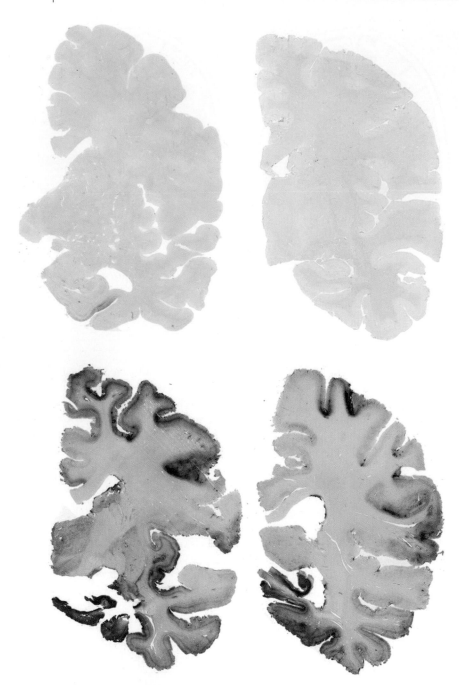

Figure 3.4 Coronal views of frontotemporal cortex in a normal brain (upper slides) and an age-matched American footballer who died of CTE. Note volume loss and characteristic immunohistochemical brown staining of Tau protein in the cortical mantle particularly in the sulcal depths and mesial temporal regions. Slides courtesy of Dr Ann McKee

attempts. It may be expedient to use a simple airway adjuncts with bag-mask ventilation, oxygenation and rapid transfer to the nearest appropriate facility ('scoop and run').

Protection of the cervical spine is mandatory in all immediate head injury management. Cervical stabilisation in a neutral position should be maintained with a semi-rigid collar, blocks and tapes. Spinal injury must be assumed in the unconscious athlete. Helmets should be removed with caution and is usually performed by two skilled personnel. Airway protection and immediate life-threatening injuries take precedence over a potential spinal injury.

In the stable breathing athlete, the most important consideration is to identify neurosurgical-type injury needing referral to hospital.

There is a number of urgent signs to watch for listed in SCAT3 (Figure 3.1). The Glasgow Coma Scale, a test of eye opening, verbal response and motor response, has merit however clinical judgement and experience are paramount. Tests of higher cortical function, eye movement and balance give more subtle and earlier clues to abnormality. Brain haemorrhage is notoriously obscured by adrenaline, and it is useful to allow a period of calm before starting the neurological examination. The lucent period of extradural haemorrhage is another pitfall.

All suspected concussions should be immediately removed from play and not return. Once ABC and neurosurgical issues are excluded, an assessment of concussion should be made using SCAT3. This covers a broad range of motor and cognitive brain functions and is much more discriminatory than tests restricted to orientation (what day?) or long-term memory (what's my name?). The five questions of Maddocks are a helpful screening tool (Figure 3.1).

Return-to-play

An athlete should not return-to-play or training until completely symptom free. This is best assessed by a medical doctor emotionally detached from the team or player. The CDC and American Academy of Neurology provide a constructive teaching video on this topic (www.cdc.gov/concussion/HeadsUp/clinicians).

The return-to-play section on SCAT3 provides an example of a six-stage graded-exercise programme (Figure 3.1). The athlete must be at least 24 h symptom free at each stage before progressing to the next (Figure 3.1).

There is a healthy culture in sport to push athletes beyond their perceived physical and mental abilities. One downside is that athletes sometimes underreport symptoms they fear might exclude them from participation or delay return-to-play. This author finds it helpful to explain to teams that (i) brain function is the primary determinant of athletic skill and performance and (ii) that playing through an unhealed concussion can delay recovery time, increase risk of recurrent concussion (especially within 10 days) and is rarely associated with second impact syndrome. The author also uses this opportunity to explain the long-term association with recurrent head injury and neurodegeneration (CTE). Head injury is sometimes associated with hypothalamo pituitary axis dysfunction, usually transient. Posttraumatic hypopituitarism can mimic physical and neuropsychiatric morbidity seen in concussed athletes especially those with coexisting loss of libido, amenorrhoea and excessive physical tiredness. Endocrine studies are required in such patients.

Many teams, schools and universities establish baseline pre-season neuropsychological scores for athletes. After concussion, the player must repeat the test and match pre-season scores. The commercially available ImPACT neurocognitive test is the most ubiquitous (www.impacttest.com). This 30-min computerised test evaluates multiple brain domains including memory, processing speed and reaction time. However, tests such as ImPACT and SCAT3 are not stand-alone measures, and there is no 'normal score' or cut-off to allow return-to-play or obviate assessment by a medical doctor.

Chronic traumatic encephalopathy

In 1928, the pathologist Harrison Martland observed that 'fight fans and promoters have recognised a peculiar condition occurring among prize fighters which, in ring parlance, they speak of as punch drunk'. This is now called chronic traumatic encephalopathy (CTE). CTE pathology is only seen in individuals exposed to recurrent brain injury. It is caused by the abnormal intraneuronal accumulation of aggregated proteins such as hyperphosphorylated Tau and TDP-43. Brain areas topographically associated with concussion are selectively vulnerable, and the symptoms of CTE reflect the neuroanatomical distribution at autopsy (amygdala,

thalamus, diencephalon, caudate, hippocampus, orbitofrontal cortex). Figure 3.4 shows CTE pathology in the brain of a deceased American footballer. The brown material is immunohistochemical staining for abnormal Tau protein.

CTE typically presents in the 40–60 age range, that is, after the athlete has retired from sport. Early symptoms tend to be psychological such as apathy, depression, impulsivity, substance abuse, breakdown in social and family relationships. Later, harder neurological signs emerge including amnesia (especially new memory acquisition), slurred speech, gait unsteadiness and parkinsonism. The most cited study, performed in professional boxers (careers 1930–1950), reported a prevalence of 17%.

Conventional imaging techniques such as CT and MRI only demonstrate late neurodegenerative changes such as significant brain atrophy. Another late radiological finding is the presence of a cavity between the two leaflets of the septum pellucidum (cavum septi pellucidi) famously depicted in the film Rocky V (Figure 3.5). This can also be a normal variant creating return-to-play dilemmas especially in boxing. It is hoped that newer techniques such as in vivo radio labelling of brain Tau protein will enable the ante-mortem diagnosis of CTE.

The Professional Fighters Brain Health Study is a large ongoing longitudinal study focusing on neurocognitive decline in boxers.

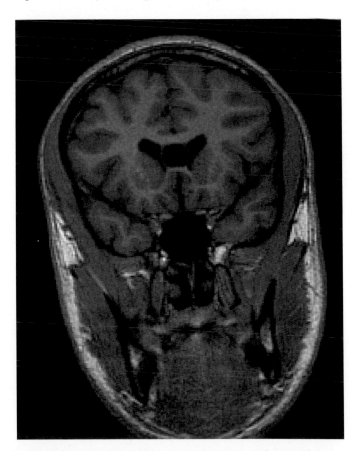

Figure 3.5 This coronal T1 MRI brain scan demonstrates the central cystic structure known as Cavum Septi Pellucidi. CSP is more common in professional boxers and may arise from repeated trauma/fenestration of the membrane or as a consequence of ex vacuo dilation. However, CSP can be a normal developmental variation. This creates clinical dilemmas when found incidentally especially in young amateur boxers

Preliminary data indicate clear correlations between neuronal loss and the number of years in boxing. For example, after 5 years, boxers show an average 1% reduction in caudate volume per additional year of fighting. Similar studies are needed in high-risk sports such as rugby and American football.

It is unclear if CTE is caused by a small number of serious brain hits, frequent sub-concussive hits or both. Genetic variation in genes such as tau and APOE4 may convey increased susceptibility. CTE has no known treatment or cure.

Head injury prevention

Helmets reduce serious face and head injury in high-velocity impact sports such as cycling, skiing and motor racing. There are similar benefits in sports using high-velocity balls. In contrast, helmets have not reduced concussion rates in most field sports like football. Helmets are particularly unhelpful for angular acceleration impact and may worsen torque. Helmets should be well fitted, bear international safety-standard stickers (e.g. ASTM, GPSR, CPSC) and be replaced regularly.

One challenge is the laboratory design of helmets that accurately model real-life concussive forces. A noteworthy example is Head Impact Telemetry (HIT). Many factors confound such as CSF, relative neck strength and how well athletes 'brace' themselves before impact. Helmets may increase head injury in other players when used as weapons, for example, 'leading with the head'. Mouthguards prevent dental and facial injury but not concussion rates.

Neck muscle strengthening and improved anticipatory neck muscle activation may modify impact forces transmitted directly to the brain, for example, reduce head twisting (angular acceleration) from a left hook in boxing. Contracting neck musculature increases the effective mass of the head, and in biomechanical terms it may disperse the energy of impact across the whole body. However, this is theoretical and unproven.

Rule change is important. For example, after the introduction of helmets in Irish Hurling, the proportion of injured players suffering a head injury went from 51% to 35%. Similarly, ice hockey benefited from body-checking rule changes. Streets with bicycle lanes have 40% fewer crashes ending in death or serious injury.

Culture change and improved player/coach awareness are also important, for example, spectators and TV commentators should be discouraged from applauding players who return to the pitch after sustaining a head injury. A major challenge facing all impact sports is to minimise concussion and CTE risk without losing the essence of the game.

Further reading

Giza, C.C. & Difiori, J.P. (2011) Pathophysiology of sports-related concussion: an update on basic science and translational research. *Sports Health*, **3**, 46–51.

Giza, C.C., Kutcher, J.S., Ashwal, S. *et al.* (2013) Summary of evidence-based guideline update: evaluation and management of concussion in sports: report of the Guideline development committee of the American Academy of Neurology. *Neurology*, **80**, 2250–7.

Martland, H.S. (1928) Punch drunk. *JAMA*, **91**, 1103–1107.

McCrory, P., Meeuwisse, W.H., Aubry, M. *et al.* (2013) Consensus statement on concussion in sport: the 4th International Conference on Concussion in Sport held in Zurich, November 2012. *British journal of Sports Medicine*, **47**, 250–8.

McKee, A.C., Stein, T.D., Nowinski, C.J. *et al.* (2013) The spectrum of disease in chronic traumatic encephalopathy. *Brain*, **136**, 43–64.

Roberts, A.H. (1969) *Brain Damage in Boxers: A Study of the Prevalence of Traumatic Encephalopathy Among Ex-Professional Boxers*. Pitman Medical Scientific Publications, London.

Roth, T.L., Nayak, D., Atanasijevic, T., Koretsky, A.P., Latour, L.L. & McGavern, D.B. (2014) Transcranial amelioration of inflammation and cell death after brain injury. *Nature*, **505**, 223–8.

Russell, W.R. (1932) Cerebral involvement in head injury. *Brain*, **55**, 549–603.

CHAPTER 4

Injury of the Face and Jaw

Keith R. Postlethwaite

Newcastle upon Tyne NHS Hospitals Trust, Newcastle upon Tyne, UK

OVERVIEW

- Although interpersonal violence is the most common cause of facial injury, sports, especially the contact sports also are often associated with facial injury. Recent studies have shown that the incidence is increasing.

- The type of facial injury that can occur during sporting activities varies from simple cuts and abrasions or minor dental injury to severely comminuted facial fractures. The latter may be associated with head and cervical spine injury. Initial attention should focus on the airway and control of bleeding.

- Injuries received often relate to the mechanism of injury, and a good history form the patient or witnesses is important for guiding clinical examination. Accurate diagnosis will aid effective initial treatment and appropriate specialist referral.

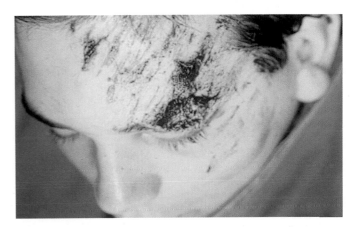

Figure 4.1 Extensive contaminated wound of forehead requiring thorough debridement and repair

Soft tissue injuries

Abrasions

Simple abrasions when contaminated require thorough cleaning and debridement to prevent infection and ugly pigmentation. This latter most commonly occurs when the abrasion is due to contact with a tarmacadum surface. Although simple debridement of superficial abrasions is possible, when large areas are involved, or where there is gross contamination, treatment may require local or sometimes general anaesthesia. Antibiotic prescription should also be considered (Figure 4.1).

Haematomas

These often settle spontaneously and rarely require drainage. However, blunt injury to the ear may result in a subperichondrial haematoma, which may result in cartilage deformity (cauliflower ear). Such haematomas should be drained either by needle aspiration or by a small incision, and a pressure dressing should be carefully applied.

Nasal septal haematomas again require evacuation to prevent necrosis of the underlying cartilage.

ABC of Sports and Exercise Medicine, Fourth Edition.
Edited by Gregory P. Whyte, Mike Loosemore and Clyde Williams.
© 2015 John Wiley & Sons, Ltd. Published 2015 by John Wiley & Sons, Ltd.

Very occasionally, large haematomas undergo liquefaction and exhibit fluctuance. If they fail to absorb after a period of 7–10 days, then drainage can be helpful.

Lacerations

Again, these should be thoroughly debrided and antibiotics be prescribed when there has been gross contamination. Thought should also be given to the need for tetanus prophylaxis.

When these are small, superficial and in uncomplicated areas of the face, accurate suturing under local anaesthesia using fine instruments and 5/0 or 6/0 monofilament nylon is appropriate. Very superficial wounds can sometimes be effectively treated with adhesive tapes (Steristrips).

Deeper lacerations will require resorbable subcutaneous sutures, such as Polyglactin (Vicryl), to approximate the skin edges prior to the placement of skin sutures. Skin sutures can be covered in a polyantibiotic ointment (Chloramycetin or Polyfax) to prevent infection and to aid their removal at 5–7 days.

Care should be taken with small puncture wounds, which may represent the entry point of a foreign body and will, therefore, require radiographic examination and possibly exploration.

It is important to check facial nerve function as lacerations involving sectioning of nerve branches should be urgently referred for microsurgical repair (Figure 4.2). Facial nerve function should

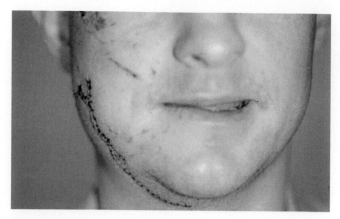

Figure 4.2 Laceration with severing of the cervical branch of the facial nerve

be checked systematically by asking the patient to look upwards or frown (frontalis branch), screw up the eyes (zygomaticotemporal), twitch the nose (buccal) and purse the lips (mandibular and cervical).

Shaving the eyebrow prior to suturing of lacerations is not recommended as it can lead to misalignment and also problems of regrowth.

Intraoral lacerations can be difficult to suture due to problems of adequate access and are probably best referred to a maxillofacial unit (Box 4.1).

Dental injury

Injury to the mouth may cause soft tissue injury and can often be associated with dental injury, teeth may be fractured, mobilised, subluxed or avulsed.

Fracturing of the teeth may involve exposure of the sensitive dentine or dental pulp, which can be extremely sensitive and painful. Such teeth require appropriate dressing by a dental surgeon.

Mobilised teeth require splinting and thorough dental evaluation to exclude fracture of the root and to monitor vitality.

Subluxation (displacement) of teeth requires repositioning usually under local anaesthesia and splinting for 7–10 days.

Avulsed teeth may be successfully re-implanted although inappropriate first aid will adversely affect the prognosis; success depends on correct initial treatment (Box 4.2).

Prevention of dental injury by the use of correctly fitted mouth guards should be mandatory in all contact sports.

Box 4.1 **Lacerations requiring specialist referral**

- Lacerations involving the lip vermilion, eyelids and lacrimal apparatus
- Be aware of nerve injuries; check facial nerve function
- Parotid duct injury
- Where there is tissue loss or full thickness laceration of the lips
- Lacerations involving the cartilage of the ear or nose
- Intraoral mucosal lacerations

Box 4.2 **Management of avulsed teeth**

- If the tooth is successfully retrieved, hold the crown, **not** the root, to avoid damaging the periodontal ligament remnants.
- Gently wash the tooth under cold tap water and, if possible, replace in the socket and retain it in this position by gently biting on a gauze or clean handkerchief.
- If this is not possible, or when there is danger of inhalation, then transport the tooth in milk or isotonic fluid if this is available.
- When avulsed teeth or fragments are not accounted for, and when there has been loss of consciousness, then the possibility of inhalation should be excluded by chest X-ray.
- Refer for further specialist treatment.

Maxillofacial fractures

Such injuries should always be suspected when there has been any facial trauma. If there is any doubt, the referral for specialist advice should be made. Be aware that facial fractures may be associated with head and cervical spine injury (Figure 4.3).

The facial skeleton is divided into thirds (Figure 4.4) to aid systematic examination. Fractures of the nasal bones, cheekbone (zygoma) and mandible are the most common facial bony injury occurring in sport.

A general examination of the face should be carried out and should include a visual inspection, looking for deformity and asymmetry. This is aided by cleaning blood from the face. The facial skeleton should then be palpated, looking for areas of tenderness and possible bony steps, most commonly felt around the orbital margins. Areas of facial paraesthesia may often indicate the presence of fractures due to damage of the various branches of the trigeminal nerve as they pass through bony canals.

Nasal fractures

These may be associated with nasal bleeding that usually responds to local measures, such as the application of pressure, or occasionally nasal packing with Vaseline ribbon gauze. When there is prolonged or excessive bleeding, this may indicate more extensive facial bony injury. On occasions, Foley catheters or Brighton's balloons may be required as postnasal packs.

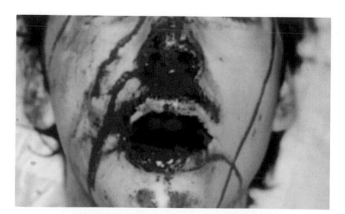

Figure 4.3 Patient with mid-face fractures; there was mobility of the maxilla

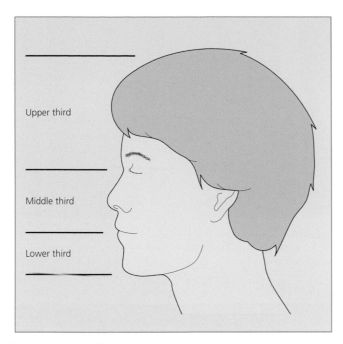

Figure 4.4 The facial thirds

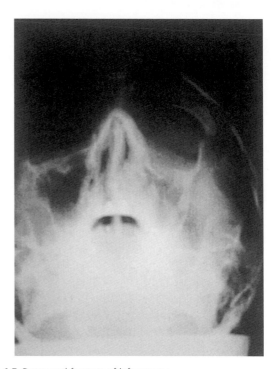

Figure 4.5 Depressed fracture of left zygoma

When seen immediately following the injury, deformity of the nose may be apparent but the rapid onset of swelling often masks this. Surgical treatment usually involves a closed manipulation of the fracture and application of a nasal splint. This treatment may be carried out immediately, but is often delayed for 7–10 days to allow swelling to settle. In some instances, late surgical intervention is indicated to correct deviation of the septal cartilage that is fractured and deviated, causing blockage of the nasal airway.

Zygomatic (cheekbone) fractures

Fractures of the zygomatic bones (Figure 4.5) result in flattening of the affected side and facial asymmetry, that is, again, often masked by swelling. Injury to the infraorbital nerve causing a characteristic area of facial numbness invariably occurs with fractures involving the zygomatic body (Figure 4.6).

As the zygoma forms both the lateral and inferior orbital walls, there is often associated injury to the eye and the periorbital tissues. The most frequent features seen are subconjunctival echymosis, blurring of vision or diplopia. When the zygomatic arch is fractured, there may be limitation of mouth opening due to the depressed arch impinging on the underlying temporalis muscle at its insertion to the coronoid process of the mandible.

Radiographic evaluation is carried out with occipitomental and submentovertex views to confirm the presence of a fracture and the degree of displacement.

Treatment involves open reduction and internal fixation with small bone plates (Figure 4.7).

Internal orbital fractures

These are more commonly known as blowout fractures and usually involve the orbital floor and occasionally the medial wall. A blowout

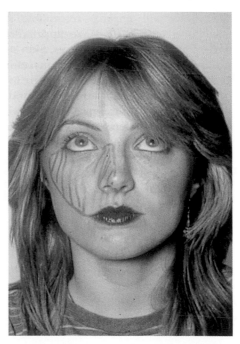

Figure 4.6 Area of numbness associated with infraorbital nerve injury

fracture should be suspected in any injury that involves a blow to the orbital area. They may be difficult to diagnose clinically and are commonly missed. The main features seen are diplopia, with 'tethering' of the affected eye, usually to upward or lateral gaze (Figure 4.8), together with paraesthesia as a result of injury to the infraorbital nerve in its bony canal. Additionally, eye movement may be painful.

A sunken appearance (enophthalmos) of the eye may be a late feature, but is often initially masked by periorbital swelling.

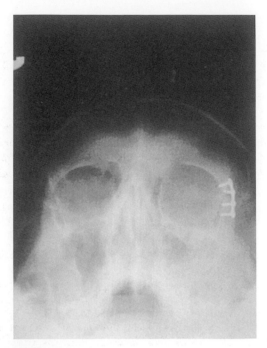

Figure 4.7 Reduction and internal fixation of fracture (right)

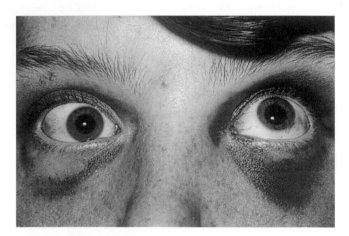

Figure 4.8 Diplopia – tethering of the right eye to upward gaze indicates a blowout fracture

Investigation usually involves a CT scan, which, as well as confirming the fracture, provides information to the site and the extent of the defect (Figure 4.9).

Treatment

All cases should undergo maxillofacial and ophthalmic assessment prior to treatment, which may involve freeing of the trapped tissue and repair of the defect to restore the contour of the orbit.

Mandibular fractures

The mandible is a horseshoe-shaped bone, and fractures often occur bilaterally. They also occur at points of weakness, the condylar neck being the most common site. Pain and difficulty in occluding the

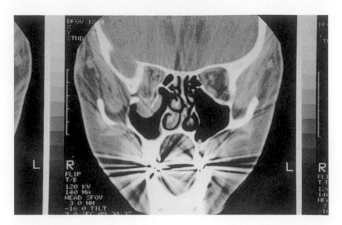

Figure 4.9 Coronal computed tomography scan confirms a blowout fracture of the right orbital floor with prolapse of tissue from the orbit into the underlying maxillary sinus

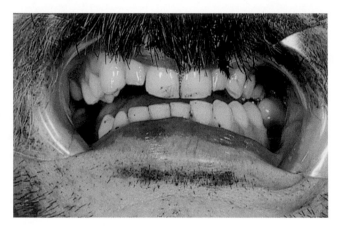

Figure 4.10 Patient with displaced middle-third facial fracture and associated

teeth are an indication of mandibular fracture. Due to damage to the mandibular nerve within its bony canal, paraesthesia of the lower lip on the affected side is often seen.

Bony steps are not easily palpable extraorally apart from grossly displaced fractures. However, intraoral examination may be more helpful in revealing obvious steps in the lower dental arch or a deranged bite (Figure 4.10), together with mucosal bruising and lacerations.

Treatment usually involves open reduction and internal fixation with small plates applied to the bone surface, most commonly via an intraoral approach.

Fractures of the middle third of face

Middle-third facial fractures are usually seen following high-velocity injuries or, on occasions, particularly violent assaults, they are not commonly seen following sporting injury, but nonetheless should always be considered in trauma to the face. They should be suspected especially when there is derangement of the dental occlusion, palpable bony steps, along the infraorbital margin, facial sensory disturbance and nasal bleeding.

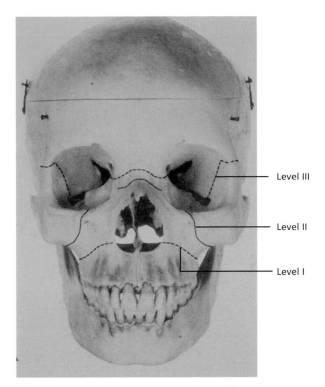

Level III

Level II

Level I

Figure 4.11 Le Fort fractures malocclusion (deranged bite)

Middle-third fractures are also associated with the mobility of the maxilla, which may be seen when the upper teeth are grasped and pressure applied.

The fractures may be classified using the Le Fort description. Fractures at the II or III levels may involve a CSF rhinorrhoea (Figure 4.11).

Summary

Soft tissue injury

- Facial and intraoral lacerations may require specialist referral.
- Be aware of underlying nerve injuries (check facial nerve function).

Dental injury

- If the tooth is successfully retrieved and complete, hold the crown, NOT the root, to avoid damaging the periodontal ligament remnants. The earliest replacement in the socket is vital to success.
- If required, transport should only be in an isotonic solution if available, milk, or the patient's own saliva.

Facial bony injury

- In all facial trauma with or without significant soft tissue injury, underlying bony injury should always be suspected with early referral for specialist advice if in any doubt.
- Following such injury, it is recommended that contact sport should be avoided for a period of 6–8 weeks.

Further reading

Crow, R. (1991) Diagnosis and management of sports-related injuries to the face. *Dental Clinics of North America*, **35**, 719–732.

Emshoff, R. *et al.* (1997) Trends in the incidence and cause of sport-related mandibular fractures. *Journal of Oral and Maxillofacial Surgery*, **55**, 585–592.

Rowe, N.L. & Williams, J.W. (eds) (1994) *Maxillofacial Injuries*. Churchill Livingstone, Edinburgh.

CHAPTER 5

Eye Injuries in Sport

Caroline J. MacEwen

Ophthalmology, University of Dundee, Dundee, UK

OVERVIEW

- Eye injuries caused by sporting activities are often serious; the most frequent sports to cause serious eye injury in the United Kingdom being football, the racket sports, rugby and hockey
- When assessing an injury, be aware of the circumstances and the type of injury suffered (e.g. blunt, sharp), as this influences the type and extent of injury sustained
- Examine the eye systematically with a good light – but do not force open swollen eyelids
- Players need to see clearly to perform well – know the method of optical correction for the 25% who have a refractive error as this may affect any injury – glasses, contact lenses, refractive surgery
- Refer immediately to a specialist opinion if a serious eye injury is suspected or if the player proves difficult to examine
- Prevention is better than cure – encourage safe play and the use of appropriate, well-fitted protective eye wear

---

Introduction

The majority of sport-associated eye injuries are superficial, involving only the external eye or surrounding tissues; however, there is risk of intra-ocular damage with potentially sight-threatening consequences in a significant minority. Approximately, 75% of sport-associated eye injuries are severe enough to require follow-up or hospital admission. Most of these injuries are entirely preventable.

Sports associated with ocular trauma

There is a close relationship between the sport being played and the risk and type of ocular injury; sports physicians need to familiarise themselves with their own sport. Close body contact, high-speed flying balls and wielding implements are risk factors for injury. Frequency of injury depends, largely, on regional and national

popularity; baseball is the commonest cause of sporting eye injury in America, hurling in Ireland and football in the United Kingdom.

The risk of injury is graded, depending on the sport being played.

Low risk

Low-velocity sports played on an individual basis, without the use of implements or balls, comprise the low-risk group. Sports such as running, cycling and swimming are in this group.

High risk

Sports that use rapidly moving balls, employ sticks and rackets or involve any degree of body contact carry a relatively high risk of injury. Such sports include the racket sports (squash, tennis and badminton), soccer, rugby, cricket and hockey.

Very high risk

The combat sports, such as boxing and karate, by their very nature comprise a very high-risk group for serious eye injuries.

Prevention and protection

It is recognised that >90% of sport-associated eye injuries are predictable and therefore avoidable. Prevention, which is vastly superior to treatment, is a priority in all sports. Strategies include the following:

- Education: teaching about the risks of injury and encouraging safe play by embedding this in coaching and training.
- Regulation: ensuring that the rules of play are in the interest of eye safety, for example, high sticks rule in hockey.
- Screening: for high-risk groups, screening is performed to prevent those with high-risk ocular conditions (e.g. high myopia, previous retinal detachment or intra-ocular surgery) or those who would be rendered visually disabled if injured (e.g. players with only one useful eye) from participating in very high-risk combat sports.
- Protection: wearing protective eyewear. British standard eye protectors are available for many sports – clear, light polycarbonate material that is fog and scratch proof (Figure 5.1), and may have a prescription incorporated into the lenses to ensure good vision. These must be tailored to the individual sport and be *fitted properly*.

ABC of Sports and Exercise Medicine, Fourth Edition.
Edited by Gregory P. Whyte, Mike Loosemore and Clyde Williams.
© 2015 John Wiley & Sons, Ltd. Published 2015 by John Wiley & Sons, Ltd.

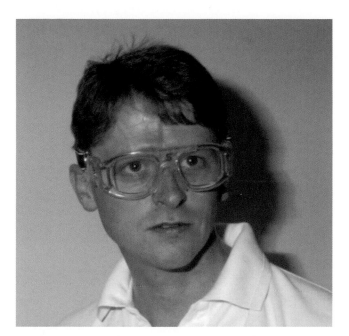

Figure 5.1 Eye protectors should be made of one-piece polycarbonate, fitted carefully and fixed firmly to the head

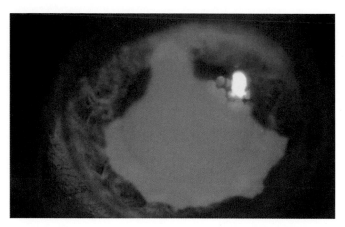

Figure 5.2 Corneal abrasion stained with fluorescein and illuminated with a blue light

Spectrum of injury

Superficial blunt trauma

The majority of all sporting eye injuries are caused by balls or collisions with other players and are, therefore, blunt in nature. The most common effects of blunt trauma include the following.

- Periorbital contusion or 'black eye' – although not a serious injury, this may cause tense eyelid swelling that prevents adequate examination of the underlying globe. It is not recommended to force the lids open as this may exacerbate any associated intra-ocular damage.
- Retro-bulbar haemorrhage – this is a rare complication of blunt ophthalmic trauma that may lead to irreversible visual loss caused by compression of the optic nerve in the orbit. This requires *urgent* orbital decompression. The clinical features are of proptosis, reduced eye movements, rapid reduction in vision and pain.
- Subconjunctival haemorrhage – easily recognised as a diffuse, uniform, bright red area covering some or all of the white of the eye, commonly occurs in association with a black eye.
- Corneal abrasion – the corneal epithelium is disrupted or removed by a direct blow causing an acutely painful corneal abrasion (Figure 5.2).

Blowout fractures

Blowout fractures occur when the eye is struck with significant blunt force – commonly a ball or a fist – and the intra-orbital pressure rises abruptly so that the floor of the orbit 'blows out' into the maxillary antrum. This may be accompanied by prolapse of the inferior orbital contents causing:

- enophthalmos – in the acute phase this is not evident due to swelling and bruising

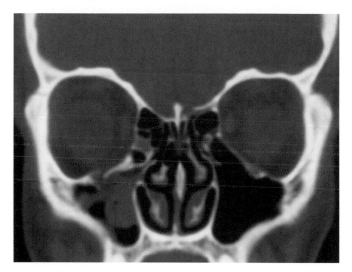

Figure 5.3 Computed tomogram showing a blowout fracture of the orbital floor – note the fracture in the floor with a drop of haemorrhage into the maxillary antrum

- infra-orbital anaesthesia
- double vision

The diagnosis is clinical, but CT scans (Figure 5.3) are required if surgery is considered necessary, usually for persistent diplopia (Figure 5.4).

Intra-ocular blunt trauma

Severe blunt injuries may cause damage to the intra-ocular contents:

- Hyphaema – Bleeding into the anterior chamber (hyphaema) implies that significant intra-ocular trauma has occurred and urgent specialist attention is required (Figure 5.5).
- Retinal tear – predisposes to a retinal detachment.
- Vitreous haemorrhage – caused by damage to retinal vessels.
- Commotio retinae – traumatic oedema of the sensory retina can be extensive and, if the macular area is involved, carries a poor prognosis for visual recovery (Figure 5.6).

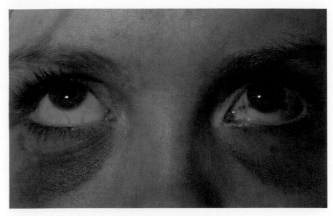

Figure 5.4 Patient unable to elevate left eye due to blowout fracture – note small subconjunctival haemorrhage and periorbital bruising

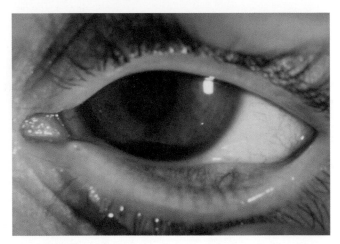

Figure 5.5 Hyphaema – level of blood visible within the anterior chamber

- Choroidal ruptures – these usually occur in the macular area, leading to considerable reduction in central vision (Figure 5.7).
- Rupture of the globe – rare, but may be the result of severe blunt trauma; the vision is dramatically reduced and there is severe subconjunctival bleeding and swelling. There may be a watery discharge from the eye.

Small foreign particles

Small pieces of foreign material, such as dust or grit, are often blown or flicked onto the eye during any outdoor activity. These particles may remain on the cornea causing intense pain. In some instances, they settle under the upper lid, as sub-tarsal foreign bodies, and rub up and down scratching the front of the eye as the lids open and close. Foreign bodies that penetrate the eye are rare in sport.

Penetrating injuries

Penetrating injuries due to rackets, sticks, fingers or fish hooks entering the globe are fortunately rare, as this type of injury tends to have a poorer prognosis (Figure 5.8). They should be suspected if the anterior chamber appears shallower or if the pupil is irregular on the injured side. Multiple intra-ocular structures may be affected, resulting in a poor visual outcome.

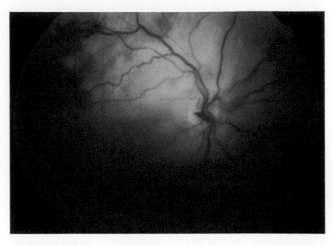

Figure 5.6 Area of commotion retina – pallor of the superior retina with the associated retinal haemorrhage

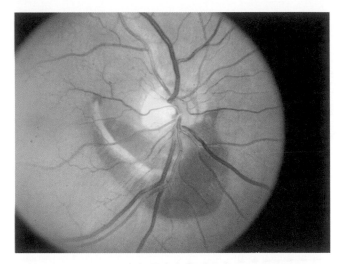

Figure 5.7 Pale crescent-shaped choroidal rupture surrounded by retinal haemorrhage

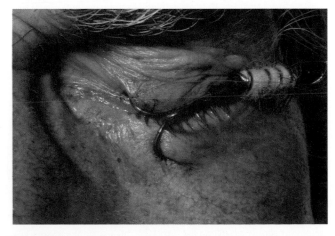

Figure 5.8 Fish hook injuries may be responsible for penetrating eye injuries

Burns

Skiers and climbers who do not use UV protectors are susceptible to 'snow blindness' due to ultraviolet light burns causing corneal de-epithelialisation. Chemical burns are rare.

Assessment and first aid

Attendance by medical and optometric staff at sports events can be anything from non-existent to fully comprehensive, with the state-of-the-art equipment at international events where emphasis is placed on optimal visual correction as well as on the initial assessment of eye injuries. Basic equipment assists examination (Box 5.1) and all injured eyes should be reviewed in a systematic manner using a good light (Box 5.2). There should be a low threshold for onward referral to a specialised unit.

The role of the attending doctor at a sports event is to

- determine whether or not an eye injury is serious (Box 5.3);
- treat minor injuries;
- sanction return to the field if considered appropriate.

Suspicion of a retro-bulbar haemorrhage should instigate an emergency referral to the nearest emergency department for a lateral cantholysis to permit orbital decompression and thus prevent permanent visual loss.

Box 5.1 Useful 'touchline' equipment for ocular assessment

- Good pen torch
- Fluorescein eye drops (single use)
- Local anaesthetic eye drops (e.g. proxymetacaine – single use)
- Cotton buds
- Broad spectrum antibiotic ointment
- Eye pad and clear shield
- Ophthalmoscope

Box 5.2 Method of examination

- Check vision (count fingers, read print or signposts) or ask about subjective change
- Fields of vision to confrontation – assess four quadrants in each eye
- Examine the eye using a good light in a systematic manner:
- periorbital region – palpate and observe
- external eye – conjunctiva; cornea; sclera (fluorescein drops)
- intra-ocular examination – anterior chamber; pupil size, shape and reaction; posterior segment
- Examine eye movements and ask about diplopia

Box 5.3 Indicators of a serious injury

- Reduced vision – subjectively or objectively
- Significant pain
- Tense orbital swelling and/or proptosis
- Hyphaema
- Abnormal pupil shape or function
- Marked subconjunctival haemorrhage or swelling
- Chemical material has entered the eye
- Diplopia in any position of gaze

Surface examination of the eye can be supplemented with a drop of fluorescein, which will assist by staining a corneal foreign body or abrasion bright green. Corneal abrasions are extremely painful, and it is unlikely that play will be resumed if one is sustained. Similarly, corneal foreign bodies will lead to suspension of play and it is not appropriate for these to be removed on the touchline. Topical antibiotic eye ointment should be instilled and a firm pad applied for those with a superficial eye injury. The upper eyelid should be everted using a cotton bud, and any foreign material sitting under the lid should be swept off. More diffuse conjunctival material, such as mud, is best removed by irrigating the eye with sterile saline. Contact lens wearers should have the lens removed from the affected eye. Instillation of local anaesthetic assists these treatments.

Hyphaema may be evident as a level of blood within the anterior chamber (Figure 5.5) but, in the acute phase, may be evident as a cloudy anterior chamber with a hazy appearance to the iris.

The pupils should be equal, round and react to light; any irregularity should be considered a sign of intra-ocular damage.

Chemical irritants should be washed out of the eye immediately and copiously before transfer to hospital, and during transport the eye should be covered with a pad or plastic shield.

Any player with a suspected serious injury should be transferred promptly to the nearest ophthalmology unit for specialist assessment and attention with the eye protected by a shield and the head immobilised.

Visual correction

Twenty-five per cent of all sportspeople require some form of refractive correction, and the method required and chosen may affect the type and severity of injury sustained. People who are short-sighted have large eyes, which are more susceptible to retinal damage, and this risk is not eliminated by refractive surgery. Refractive correction may be of the following forms:

Spectacles

This is the simplest method that provides the best corrected vision and therefore should be used for high-acuity sports, for example shooting. Not suitable for contact sports as may damage self or opponent.

Contact lenses

Soft lenses – very large diameter, lenses are relatively stable in the eye and are best for contact and combat sports.

Hard lenses may break in the eye and cause ocular damage.

Refractive surgery

Incisional surgery is rarely performed now, but there are still people who have had this surgery. This causes a weak eye and may have disastrous consequences due to globe rupture (Figure 5.9).

Surface-based laser surgery (photorefractive keratectomy) is relatively safe and does not weaken the cornea.

Intra-corneal LASIK is the mainstay of refractive corrective surgery, but is not compatible with contact sports for 6–12 months as there is a risk of the superficial flap becoming dislodged and lost.

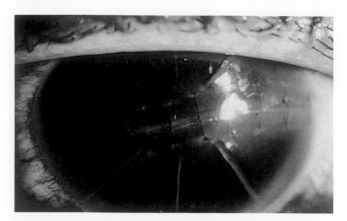

Figure 5.9 Repair of cornea after incisional refractive surgery. The eye had been struck by a squash racket causing rupture of one of the radial refractive incisions (sutured). Any ocular surgery wound is susceptible to rupture. Reproduced courtesy of Dr G. Crawford, Perth, Western Australia

It is vital to be aware of the current and past spectacle requirement, method of correction and any previous ocular surgery for all players.

Arrange immediate referral to hospital if there is any doubt about the severity or nature of the injury.

Further reading

Barr, A., MacEwen, C.J., Desai, P. & Baines, P.S. (2000) Ocular sports injuries – the current picture. *British Journal of Sports and Exercise Medicine*, **34**, 456–8.

Loran, D.F.C. & MacEwen, C.J. (eds) (1995) *A Textbook of Sports Vision*. Butterworth Heinemann, Oxford.

MacEwen, C.J. (1986) Sport-associated eye injuries: a casualty department survey. *The British Journal of Ophthalmology*, **71**, 701–5.

Ong, H.S., Barsam, A., Morris, O.C., Siriwardena, D. & Verma, S. (2012) A Survey of Ocular Sports Trauma and the role of eye protection. *Contact Lens and Anterior Eye*, **35**, 285–87.

Vinger, P.F. (1981) Sports eye injuries; a preventable disease. *Ophthalmology*, **88**, 108–12.

Zagelbaum, B.M. (ed) (1996) *Sports Ophthalmology*. Blackwell Science, Oxford.

CHAPTER 6

Management of Injuries in Children

Julian Redhead

Emergency Medicine, Imperial College School of Medicine, London, UK

OVERVIEW

- There are specific differences in between adults and children, which must be considered when evaluating a child. Certain injuries only occur in children
- All clinicians have a responsibility to promote exercise to children
- All clinicians must be aware of potential abuse to children
- The pattern of injury is different in children when compared to adults
- All clinicians should be alert to the possibility of malignancy, even where the presentation appears to be related to an injury

---

Every human being below 18 years
— United Nations Convention on the rights of a child

'Children are not little adults' – a cliché, but never more true than for Paediatric Exercise Medicine and injuries. The examination of a child is a skill and involves observation of the child playing and interacting as well as examination of relevant systems. There are a number of significant adaptations which should be made when assessing a child and when considering the pathology of their injuries or issues.

All the Ps

Physical
Physiological
Psychological
Protection
Pathological

Physical

Children grow by a series of growth spurts and the timings of these growth spurts vary between children – although consistently, the maximum acceleration of growth occurs at puberty. This difference

ABC of Sports and Exercise Medicine, Fourth Edition.
Edited by Gregory P. Whyte, Mike Loosemore and Clyde Williams.
© 2015 John Wiley & Sons, Ltd. Published 2015 by John Wiley & Sons, Ltd.

in growth can lead to a mismatch in size between children of the same-age group and may be significant in the injury pattern of children competing in contact sports.

Growth spurts have been recognised at a time where there is a heightened risk of injury. The overall body shape changes, resulting, temporarily, in a potentially less balanced and uncoordinated child. The segmental proportions differ so that the head size becomes proportionally smaller and the limbs proportionally longer – the bone lengthening before the muscle–tendon unit. The muscle tends to increase in strength before the tendon can adapt and strengthen.

The increasing limb length and relatively poor muscle control of the limb lead to greater forces acting through movement, while the greater muscle mass before tendon adaptation leads to greater forces acting through the tendon and hence potential injuries.

The skeleton is developing, involving both linear growth and skeletal maturation (Figure 6.1). There is an orderly process of cartilage cell division, followed by the production of a matrix which then calcifies and is converted into bone. This process of endochondral ossification is occurring in the physes (growth plates), epiphyses (articular surface) and apophyses (tendon bone junction). These growth areas are susceptible to injuries and repeated stress (Figures 6.2 and 6.3).

The bones have a higher water content and lower mineral content than adults, and so the bones tend to be less brittle. The periosteum is thicker. This leads to the potential for a bone to buckle, rather than break and the characteristic greenstick or torus fracture found in children.

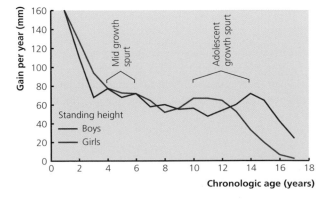

Figure 6.1 Linear growth in children. Source: Duthie RB. The Significance of Growth in Orthopedic Surgery, Clinical Orthopedics 1959; 14:7–18.

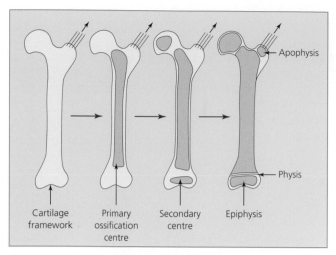

Figure 6.2 Endochondral ossification (diagram). Conversion of cartilage into bone. Source: A level 2 course national coaching foundation leads.

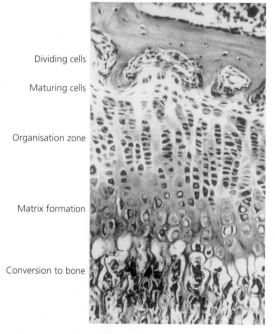

Dividing cells

Maturing cells

Organisation zone

Matrix formation

Conversion to bone

Figure 6.3 Endochondral ossification (Radiographs). Source: Ham AW, Lesson TS. HAM Histology, Pitman Medical Publishing Co. Ltd, London (a JB Lippincott company), 1961.

The bones also tend to have a better blood supply, which allows faster healing and remodelling of bone injury sites.

The young child has an ability to adapt and learn, and is the ideal time for patterns of movement, needed for specific sports to be learnt.

Physiological

Respiratory rate, heart rate and blood pressure all change during maturation, and these are indicators of the physiological changes occurring in the body.

Age (years)	Respiratory rate	Heart rate
2–5	25–30	95–140
5–12	20–25	80–120
>12	15–20	60–100

It is important to know the normal ranges for children so that abnormal parameters can be recognised. Children tend to have a large physiological reserve and can appear to be coping until sudden deterioration occurs. They have a smaller circulating blood volume and are thus more prone to hypovolaemia.

There is an increased incidence of heat exhaustion in children compared to adults.

Children

- produce more heat relative to body mass
- lower sweating capacity
- tendency to not drink enough fluids during exercise.

Psychological

The benefits of an active lifestyle are now established, and it is our responsibility as healthcare professionals to promote these. A healthy lifestyle as a child is the foundation for a similar approach in adulthood and will benefit the population as a whole.

When treating a child, attention must also be paid to the parents. They will know their child better than the treating specialist, and should be listened to. They should also be encouraged to participate in the rehabilitation of the child and in the promotion of a healthy lifestyle.

Some parents may have a negative effect on the child – the well-used example of the touchline parent, pressurising the child to succeed. However, bullying can take many forms in sport from physical to emotional, and mechanisms must be in place to recognise and eradicate this and other forms of abuse.

During development, children will mature in their ideas and personality. Sexual maturation will occur. These factors must be taken into account when integrating children of different development into sporting environments.

Children have a huge potential to learn, and so technique training should be the predominant modality. However, all training should be directed towards the child having fun and enjoying the experiences they are gaining.

Protection

All institutions involved with children should have clear policies regarding child protection and clearly identified personnel responsible for safe guarding. All suspicions should be reported and correlated with other agencies such as school nurses, general practitioners and social services.

Coaches and medical staff have a responsibility to protect the children in their care and allow them to develop in a safe but challenging environment. All should be aware of the potential types of abuse, and as medical practitioners we should be aware of the potential for non-accidental injuries and their recognition.

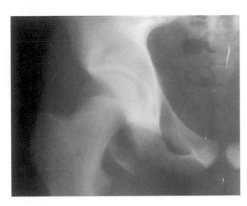

Figure 6.4 Acute bony avulsion ischium

Non-accidental injury red flags

Delay in presentation
Recurrent unexplained injury
Unusual pattern of injury
Withdrawn child
Hiding injuries

Generally, children are risk takers and do not necessarily think through the consequences of their actions. It is important to ensure that children are involved in decisions about their treatment, but explain the consequences in a way that the child will understand. Legally a child who is felt to have the necessary competence can consent to treatment, but cannot refuse a treatment, without parental consent.

Pathological

Due to these physical changes, certain injuries are more common or unique in the paediatric population. These include both acute and overuse type of injuries.

Acute injuries

Tendon–bone junctions

As described earlier, the weakest part of the link between muscles and bone is at their junction. Children will tend to have an avulsion fracture (Figure 6.4) than a muscle or tendon injury. Common sites of injury include the following:

Muscle	Attachment
Hamstring	Ischial tuberosity
Rectus femoris	Anterior inferior iliac spine
Sartorius	Anterior superior iliac spine

Management of tendon–bone junction injury

- The management can be active or conservative depending on the site and displacement of the fragment and also the age of the child.

- Many avulsion fractures of the tibial spines, for example, can be managed by manipulation into extension and then immobilisation, but others may require internal fixation.
- The outcome of these injuries should be good and even what might be seen as a significant displacement can indeed be accepted, and healing can proceed without long-term effects.

Torus and greenstick fractures

Buckle fractures or torus fractures are typically stable injuries that only require immobilisation with a splint for analgesia. Mobilisation can occur as pain allows.

Greenstick fractures are when one cortex is broken and the other is bent. These may be more unstable and require manipulation, but again heal well and may need a splint or plaster depending on site and severity.

Management of buckle and greenstick fractures

- Radiological assessment
- Appropriate immobilisation for pain relief
- Mobilisation once the fracture is pain free and has healed

Physeal injuries

These are injuries to the physeal plate; if severe, they can permanently arrest growth in part or in all of the physis (Figure 6.5). These

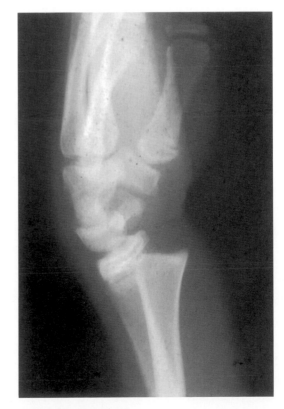

Figure 6.5 Physeal fracture of wrist

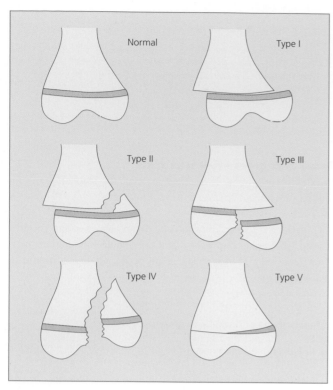

Figure 6.6 Salter–Harris classification. Salter RB, Harris WR. "Injuries involving the epiphyseal plate". Source: J Bone Joint Surg [Am] 1963; 45-A: 587–622

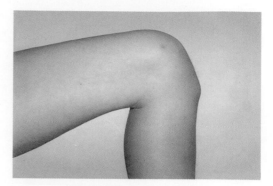

Figure 6.7 Osgood-Schlatter's disease

are common and have no equivalent in adults. The Salter–Harris classification of physeal fractures is a useful tool (Figure 6.6). Types I and II fractures have an intact physeal plate, and the prognosis is very good. Closed reduction of the fracture should ensure normal physeal growth. In types III and IV fractures, the physeal plate is disrupted, and this must be reduced anatomically. Without anatomical reduction, union of the epiphysis to the metaphysis preventing the physis growing is a risk, and asymmetrical growth can follow. This can lead to deformity that may need correcting. Type V fractures are injuries to the physeal plate and, if severe, can permanently arrest growth in part or all of the physis. These can be difficult fractures to diagnose even with X-ray.

> **Management of physeal injuries**
>
> - Early recognition and assessment of the injury
> - Anatomical reduction of the physis is needed, particularly if the fracture crosses the plate, as this often needs surgical intervention
> - Immobilisation
> - Rehabilitation
> - Careful monitoring to identify any abnormality of subsequent growth

Overuse skeletal injuries

Osteochondrosis

This term refers to a collection of disorders where there is a derangement to the normal growth of the epiphysis. The conditions are all self-limiting. The condition can affect any epiphysis and most have acquired eponyms. Generally, they are classified according to their position:

Articular	Non-articular	Physeal
Frieberg's (second metatarsal)	Osgood-Schlatter (tibial tubercle) (Figure 6.7)	Schuermann's (thoracic spine)
Kohler's (navicular)	Sever's (calcaneus)	Blount's (proximal tibia)
Kienbock's (lunate)	Sinding–Larsen–Johansson (inferior pole patella)	
Perthes (femoral head)		
Osteochondritis dissecans (varied positions))		

Identification is usually clinical and supported by radiographs where doubt exists. They often present following a growth spurt, or at times of increased activity in training or competition.

Articular osteochondrosis

These can be either a primary involvement of the articular and epiphyseal cartilage such as Frieburg's or a secondary involvement or a secondary to necrosis of the adjacent bone, such as Perthes, Kohler's or osteonecrosis dissecans (Figure 6.8).

In the upper limb, this type of condition occurs in the capitellum of the humerus and is seen in children who participate in sports such as gymnastics and those who involve compressive strains on the elbow joint. Sometimes, the whole capitellum can be affected and becomes avascular; this is termed **Panner's disease**.

The patient usually initially presents with joint pain or an effusion. This can often be mild at first and slowly progressive. In the lower limb, a limp often is present, whereas in the elbow, one of the early signs is loss of full extension to the joint due to the effusion. Pain can be progressive and may lead to locking, if the cartilage and bone fragment and a loose body forms.

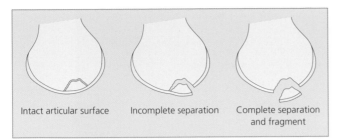

Intact articular surface   Incomplete separation   Complete separation and fragment

Figure 6.8 Osteochondritis dissecans. Epiphyseal injuries can go through different stages: from avascular segment with articular surface through segment with partial separation of fragment to complete separation of segment such that it forms a loose body

The diagnosis is made by having a suspicion from the history and on clinical examination. This can be confirmed by imaging. Radiographs usually show the involved segment, and a magnetic resonance imaging scan can also be helpful, especially in the early stages.

If the diagnosis is made early, the condition may not necessarily progress – it can heal and leave a congruous joint such that normal activities can be resumed.

Management of articular osteochondrosis injury

- In the early stages with an intact articular surface, a period of non-weight bearing may be needed if the symptoms are severe.
- Slow increase in activities can be allowed, as long as no symptoms recur. Careful follow-up is essential, with imaging, as needed, to identify the progression of healing.
- Arthroscopic assessment can often be needed if symptoms persist. With partial separation of the fragment, operative intervention may be beneficial.
- Once a loose body is diagnosed, surgical removal is necessary. Later consideration of chondral grafting techniques may be appropriate.

The natural history of healing of articular osteochondrosis may take 18 months or more. In some sports, this may curtail a patient's ability to participate and achieve.

Non-articular osteochondrosis

Diagnosis of these conditions is usually clinical. Radiographs are often misinterpreted, especially by junior doctors as demonstrating avulsion fractures.

These conditions occur most commonly at the time of the growth spurt, when the apophyses are relatively weak and the muscles relatively tight, as they grow in length less quickly than the bone. Times of increased activity in training or competition can also be a factor. Tendon bone junction injuries are recognised by point tenderness at the muscle insertion.

Management of non-articular osteochondrosis

- Careful explanation of the condition.
- Rest and restriction of activity according to levels of pain. Complete restriction of activity or immobilisation of the limb rarely required.
- Arrange training around the injury, with care not to produce an injury of a different area because of overconcentration of activity.
- Physiotherapy to address muscle balance to gently stretch the affected muscle. Care is needed not to adversely affect the condition.
- Reassurance that resolution is virtually certain but needs patience.

Physeal osteochondrosis

Scheuermann's lesions of the spine occur as a result of flexion forces acting on the anterior part of the vertebral body. The anterior growth plate is damaged and the vertebrae may become wedged, resulting in a kyphotic spinal deformity. This can occur in the thoracic and lumbar spines, and is more common in children with tight hamstrings.

Management of spinal physeal osteochondrosis

- Early radiological diagnosis
- Rest
- Careful review to identify any kyphotic deformity
- Slow, progressive activity once symptoms settle
- Gradual reintroduction of sporting activity

Stress fractures

Stress fractures of the long bones and other parts of the skeleton occur in children just as they do in adults and should be treated in the same way (Figure 6.9).

Stress fractures occur in children across virtually the whole sporting spectrum, with high incidences reported in gymnastics, cricket and rugby

A stress fracture of the **pars intra-articularis** (Figure 6.10) of the lamina of the spinal vertebra is relatively common in children, especially adolescents. The injury is caused by extension and rotational

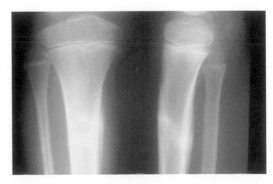

Figure 6.9 Stress fracture of the tibia in a child

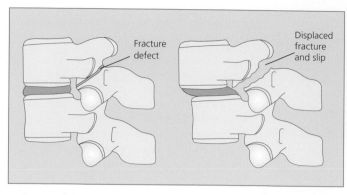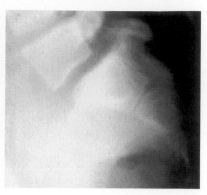

Figure 6.10 Stress fracture of the pars intra-articularis (a) and X-ray showing vertebral slip (b)

stresses, and an examination will usually demonstrate exacerbation of the pain when exerting these forces on the child back. Neurological findings would be unusual.

The defect in the lamina is initially a stress reaction and cannot be seen radiologically; bone scanning techniques or reverse gantry computed tomography scanning is needed to pick up the injury at that stage. Alternatively, pars specific magnetic resonance imaging sequences may detect these lesions and reduce radiation exposure in children.

Stress reaction to the bone can develop to form a bony defect known as spondylolysis – this can be detected on normal X-rays of the spin. Spondylolysis can develop into a forward slip of the affected vertebra on the vertebra below – a condition known as a spondylolisthesis. Prognosis generally is good, and surgical intervention is not usually needed.

Management of stress fracture

- Absolute rest from activities exacerbating pain
- Appropriate core stabilisation exercises
- Gradual reintroduction of activities

Hip pathology

A limp in a child is a common presentation to a medical practitioner. These may be associated with a specific injury; however, sometimes they will not be associated or the child/parents will correlate the limp to an injury spuriously.

Children will often report knee or thigh pain, although the pathology is in the hip joint. Examination of the hip joint should always be part of a knee examination. Restriction of internal rotation and/or abduction of the hip joint are often significant. If the child is pyrexial, an infective cause should always be excluded.

As practitioners, we need keep an open mind when considering the differential diagnosis of the limping child.

Four common causes of a limp, not related to trauma, are as follows:

Perthes

Articular osteochondrosis of the femoral head
Peak presentation in children from 4 years to about 10 years
Often presents as a painless limp
Can be bilateral
X-ray or MRI features are characteristic

Slipped femoral epiphysis

Boys affected more than girls
Correlation with obese children
Peak presentation in children from 10 to 17 years
Presents with painful limp
Can be bilateral
X-ray of the hip should confirm the diagnosis. A 'frogs leg view' may be beneficial.

Transient synovitis

This should be a diagnosis of exclusion
A causal relationship with a recent viral infection may be noticeable
Peak presentation in children less than 10 years old
Presents with painful limp X-ray will be normal, and an ultrasound should detect a joint effusion.

Septic arthritis

Can occur in any age group
Presents with a painful limp
May be pyrexial, but not necessarily
Blood tests may show evidence of infection, but not consistently
X-ray can be normal
Ultrasound will show an effusion, and an aspiration will confirm the diagnosis
Where this diagnosis is considered, the child should be cared for by an experienced clinician

Other differential diagnosis of the limping child to consider include

Juvenile rheumatoid arthritis and malignancy

Malignancy

Medical practitioners should always be aware of the possibility of childhood malignancy. Although rare, there is often a delay in diagnosis. The child or parents will often relate the beginning of symptoms to an injury.

Features in the history which may be significant for a potential diagnosis of malignancy include the following:

Night pain
Weight loss
Night sweats
Associated systemic symptoms

Any suspicion of a malignancy should mandate review by an experienced clinician.

Further reading

Caine, D., Purcell, L. & Maffulli, N. (2014) The child and adolescent athlete: a review of three potentially serious injuries. *BMC Sports Science, Medicine and Rehabilitation*, **6**, 22. doi:10.1186/2052-1847-6-22cCollection 2014. Review

Duthie, R.B. (1959) The significance of growth in orthopedic surgery. *Clinical Orthopaedics*, **14**, 7–18.

Emery, C. (2010) Injury prevention in paediatric sport-related injuries: a scientific approach. *British Journal of Sports Medicine*, **44**, 64–69. doi:10.1136/bjsm.2009.068353

Ham, A.W. & Lesson, T.S. (1961) *HAM Histology*. Pitman Medical Publishing Co. Ltd, London (a JB Lippincott company).

Pieles, G.E., Horn, R., Williams, C.A. & Stuart, A.G. (2014) Paediatric exercise training in prevention and treatment. *Archives of Disease in Childhood*, **99** (4), 380–385. doi:10.1136/archdischild-2013-303826. Epub 2013 Dec 18

Redhead, J. & Gordon, J. (2012) *Emergencies in Sports Medicine*. Oxford University Press, England.

Salter, R.B. & Harris, W.R. (1963) Injuries involving the epiphyseal plate. *The Journal of Bone and Joint Surgery. American Volume*, **45-A**, 587–622.

Weiser, P. (2012) Approach to the patient with noninflammatory musculoskeletal pain. *Pediatric Clinics of North America*, **59** (2), 471–492. doi:10.1016/j.pcl.2012.03.012. Review

CHAPTER 7

Management of Musculoskeletal Injuries in the Mature Athlete

Khan Karim[1] and Peter D. Brukner[2]

[1]Sport and Exercise Medicine, Qatar National Orthopedic and Sports medicine Hospital (ASPETAR), Doha, Qatar
[2]Sport and Exercise Medicine, Olympic Park Sports Medicine Centre, Olympic Park, Melbourne, Australia

---

OVERVIEW

In this chapter, we describe the management of musculoskeletal injuries in the mature athlete. After studying this chapter, the reader will know:

- Injury prevention and how to reduce injury risk
- Common musculoskeletal injuries
- Contributing factors to injury risk
- Management of injuries

Successful ageing through sport

The population is ageing and the number of older adults who regularly engage in physical activity is decreasing. Paradoxically, the number of older adults involved in recreational and competitive sport in the western world is increasing; the growing popularity of senior and masters sporting events around the world is testament to this. In the later years of life, maintaining regular physical activity through sports participation is associated with appreciable health and quality of life benefits.

What defines a 'mature' athlete? In some sports, such as football and basketball, 35-year-olds are considered to be approaching retirement age. In sports such as golf, players can achieve their career-best performances in their fifties. Clearly, the definition of a mature athlete depends on the sport in question. However, for simplicity and for the purpose of this chapter, a mature athlete will be defined as an individual who regularly participates in sport and is over the age of 65 years.

It is important to broadly consider the effect of ageing on an athlete's body. How does that affect the individual's ability to participate in high-level sport? Normal age-related changes in muscle strength, tendon and ligament elasticity, bone density and cartilage volume reduce an individual's peak performance over time. However, the degree of decline varies considerably between individuals. Musculoskeletal injuries can affect the confidence of the older athlete and

encourage physical inactivity. Hence, by preventing and treating injury, the sports medicine clinician can play an important role in helping older individuals maintain health and well-being. This chapter reminds the reader to consider prevention and then aims to provide sports medicine clinicians with strategies to prevent and manage musculoskeletal injuries in the mature athlete.

Injury prevention

Injury prevention is important in mature athletes because of the slower rate of healing and the negative effect that injuries can have on physical activity and mental well-being in this age group. Injury prevention strategies that clinicians should emphasise with older athletes include the following:

- The need for a proper warm-up and cool-down before and after activity
- The need to avoid abrupt changes in training frequency, duration and intensity (focus on progressive overload)
- The importance of adequate recovery between high-intensity training sessions
- The need to adjust training intensity to suit weather/environmental conditions, for example, humidity, extreme hot and cold or altitude changes
- The importance of maintaining appropriate nutritional and fluid requirements (a dietician referral may be warranted).

Musculoskeletal injuries in the mature athlete

Common musculoskeletal injuries in the mature athlete include the following:

1 Muscle strains associated with age-related muscle stiffening
2 Tendinopathies related to age-related changes in flexibility and strength of tendons as well as in degenerative changes from repetitive loading forces throughout life (particularly the rotator cuff muscles in the shoulder and the Achilles tendon)
3 Age-related articular cartilage changes, for example, osteoarthritis and degenerative tears of the menisci of the knee.

ABC of Sports and Exercise Medicine, Fourth Edition.
Edited by Gregory P. Whyte, Mike Loosemore and Clyde Williams.
© 2015 John Wiley & Sons, Ltd. Published 2015 by John Wiley & Sons, Ltd.

Table 7.1 Contributing factors to injury and decline in athletic performance in the mature athlete

- Medical history: increase in prevalent medical conditions
- Past musculoskeletal injuries
- Age-related hormonal changes
- Training errors ± loss of motivation
- Biomechanical faults associated with structural changes in joints, musculotendinous stiffness and changes in collagen

Contributing factors to musculoskeletal injuries in the mature athlete

Previous history of musculoskeletal injury is the most important risk factor for future injury. However, age-related changes such as degenerative joint diseases and/or reduced mechanical joint stability, altered proprioception, diminished vestibular function and visual impairment should also be considered risk factors for musculoskeletal injury in this population. Table 7.1 summarises contributing factors that can impair performance and musculoskeletal injury in the mature athlete.

Management

The management of acute musculoskeletal injuries in older athletes should follow a similar pathway to that of the younger athlete. The initial management of rest, ice, compression and evaluation (RICE) for acute musculoskeletal injuries applies. Note that this protocol has now been amended to include optimal loading (promoting mechanotherapy, see later), and the acronym is therefore POLICE (pain relief, optimal loading, ice, compression and elevation).

It is important to remember that musculoskeletal changes are not the only issues that the mature athlete may need to address. The judicious clinician should not forget or underestimate cardiovascular changes that impact on musculoskeletal function, changes in metabolism and immune function (which can affect recovery and healing times) and pain perception/mechanisms. Neuromuscular and central processing changes can manifest as slower reaction times, reduced postural control and potentially greater injury risk. Overall, slower recovery from injury, slower healing times, changes in sporting performance (reduction in overall force and power) will affect the management of musculoskeletal injuries in the mature athlete and may lead to reductions in participation in sports. As in any clinical setting, close discussion of goals applies (Figure 7.1).

A specific issue in the older athlete is to carefully evaluate how existing medical conditions or associated medications may influence the capacity to exercise and the safety of exercising. Medication can make exercise difficult; certain cardiovascular medications limit exercise capacity. Similarly, the patient who complains of exercise-related muscle pain may be suffering adverse effects of medication, that is, statin treatment. Full discussion of the various possible exercise associations with medication is beyond the scope of this chapter, but we recommend careful medical evaluation of older athletes who are taking multiple medications. Exercise may well be therapeutic even if there are numerous comorbidities, and there is evidence that reducing the number and the dose of medication can improve patient's quality of life in certain cases. Polypharmacy – too much medicine – is a major cause of illness and death. Clinical decisions must be made on a case-by-case basis with expert clinician assessment.

Case scenario: *Hamstring strain*

Management of a 70-year-old sprinter with a hamstring strain begins as it would in the case of a younger athlete. Is the history and physical examination consistent with an acute muscle strain? If so, careful physical examination aims to identify if the lesion is in the biceps (type 1 hamstring strain) or semimembranosus/semitendinosus (type 2 hamstring strain). The former is more likely in a sprinter. Before moving on, the diagnosis requires the clinician to rule out a complete avulsion (discussed at the bottom of this scenario).

Whether MRI is indicated depends on the overall clinical setting. Swedish expert Dr Carl Askling argues for it to help make the diagnosis accurately. However, many clinicians have successfully guided rehabilitation at all ages on clinical grounds alone.

The treatment of choice is to use standard management principles. In the older person, the progression will need to be slower and the initial loads lower. However, other criteria, that is, pain free, not tender to palpation, remain the same as in the younger athlete.

Risk of recurrence is a major concern in athletes of all ages, but there are no studies to guide us in the management of the mature athlete in this regard. Clinically, given the reduced rates of repair in mature athletes, a slower return to play, a reduction in match/race intensity upon return and attention to recovery methods (i.e. massage) are logical.

Hamstring return to play should be guided by clinical indicators – pain-free movement, full knee extension, pain-free lesion site to palpation (lack of tenderness) and the ability to progressively return to the functional sporting activities. The progression for a sprinter would be from jogging (weeks) to 'run throughs' (faster pace), 'stride throughs' (even faster) (both phases taking weeks) and then return towards full sprinting over a period of

---

'How often do you run and what distances?'

'Do you play golf regularly?'

'How long do you intend to continue competing?'

Asking the injured mature athlete these types of questions will give a clinician a sense of patient expectations for frequency of exercise and level of intensity which will help devise an appropriate management plan.

Figure 7.1 Management of musculoskeletal injuries in the mature athlete

another few weeks if all the milestones are met (as listed above, pain-free, full range of motion, and so on). Thus, a progression in a mature athlete may take 2–4 weeks longer than in an athlete in her or his twenties.

Noteworthy, if it is a complete avulsion surgery is generally not indicated as conservative management can lead to full clinical recovery.

Case scenario: *Achilles tendinopathy*

Careful localisation of the point of pain and tenderness is a key factor in the diagnosis of Achilles tendinopathy at any age. Rupture needs to be ruled out by history and the Thomson or Simmonds test. For tendinopathy, mid-Achilles pain responds more quickly and predictably than insertional Achilles tendinopathy. The reader is referred to Jill Cook's 'continuum approach' (see further reading) to managing tendinopathy and the core concept that loading is essential for tendon repair. Rest has often been tried, and this does not providing an appropriate stimulus for tendon healing. Once there has been appropriate period of 'relative rest', the older athlete may well need *more* stimulus than a younger counterpart to promote tissue healing. As in any case of tendinopathy, contributing extrinsic (e.g. load, surface) or intrinsic (biomechanics, arthropathy) needs to be considered. The role of rigid orthoses (in conjunction with shoe choice) in treatment of Achilles tendinopathy divides the clinical community, and there are few high-quality trials to guide management. Orthoses should be considered on a case-by-case basis – using the extent of abnormal biomechanics as a guide.

Case scenario: *Knee osteoarthritis*

Many older people have clinical knee osteoarthritis. Exercise should be considered a part of treatment in this condition. Thus, exercise should be encouraged for those who wish to exercise and those who do not! Let us focus on the person who is keen to exercise but finds that long running aggravates his or her knee pain.

Alternative forms of exercise that promotes joint movement but do not compress the joint as much as running often allows a mature athlete to gain the cardiovascular and mental benefits that they so crave. Biking and swimming are obvious choices and a large number of older persons riding in large pelotons are the testament to the effectiveness of this treatment. Systematic reviews of randomised trials indicate that exercise is an effective treatment for knee osteoarthritis with moderate effect size.

The question of whether either aerobic exercise or progressive resistance training influences quality of life of patients who have undergone total knee replacement remains unanswered. The clinical impression is that the benefits of exercise should include assistance in maintaining healthy weight and muscle strength in addition to systemic benefits such as cardiovascular and mental health. However, this needs to be weighed against the potential that loading the implant will lead to more rapid wear and the potential for loosening. The clinical impression among joint replacement surgeons and clinicians is that exercise activity within the guideline range has not provided evidence of accelerated deterioration.

Summary

Peak performance falls over time related to changes in muscle strength, tendon and ligament elasticity, bone density and cartilage volume. The degree of decline varies considerably between individuals; however, injury prevention is important in mature athletes because of the slower rate of healing and the negative effect that injuries can have on physical activity and mental well-being in this age group. Previous history of musculoskeletal injury is the most important risk factor for future injury; however, a range of risks should also be considered. The management of acute musculoskeletal injuries in mature athletes should follow a similar pathway to that of the younger athlete with acute injury following the POLICE approach. It is important to carefully evaluate how existing medical conditions or associated medications may influence the capacity to exercise and the safety of exercising.

Further reading

Alexandratos, K., Barnett, F. & Thomas, Y. (2012) The impact of exercise on the mental health and quality of life of people with severe mental illness: a critical review. *The British Journal of Occupational Therapy*, **75** (**2**), 48–60.

Bleakley, C.M., Glasgow, P. & MacAuley, D.C. (2012) PRICE needs updating, should we call the POLICE? *British Journal of Sports Medicine*, **46** (**4**), 220–1. doi:10.1136/bjsports-2011-090297. Epub 2011 Sep 7.

Cook, J.L. & Purdam, C.R. (2009) Is tendon pathology a continuum? A pathology model to explain the clinical presentation of load-induced tendinopathy. *British Journal of Sports Medicine*, **43** (**6**), 409–16. doi:10.1136/bjsm. 2008.051193. Epub 2008 Sep 23.

Hamilton, C.J., Swan, V.J. & Jamal, S.A. (2010) The effects of exercise and physical activity participation on bone mass and geometry in postmenopausal women: a systematic review of pQCT studies. *Osteoporosis International*, **21** (**1**), 11–23.

McAlindon, T.E., Bannuru, R.R., Sullivan, M.C. *et al.* (2014) OARSI guidelines for the non-surgical management of knee osteoarthritis. *Osteoarthritis Cartilage*, **22** (**3**), 363–88. doi:10.1016/j.joca.2014.01.003. Epub 2014 Jan 24.

McCarthy, M.M. & Hannafin, J.A. (2014) The mature athlete: aging tendon and ligament. *Sports Health*, **6**, 141–148.

Moynihan, R., Heneghan, C. & Godlee, F. (2013) Too much medicine: from evidence to action. *BMJ.*, **347**, f7141. doi:10.1136/bmj.f7141.

Onambele, G.L., Narici, M.V. & Maganaris, C.N. (2006) Calf muscle-tendon properties and postural balance in old age. *Journal of Applied Physiology*, **100** (**6**), 2048–2056.

Perraton, L.G., Kumar, S. & Machotka, Z. (2010) Exercise parameters in the treatment of clinical depression: a systematic review of randomized controlled trials. *Journal of Evaluation in Clinical Practice*, **16** (**3**), 597–604.

Siparsky, P.N., Kirkendall, D.T. & Garrett, W.E. (2014) Muscle changes in aging: understanding sarcopenia. *Sports Health*, **6** (**1**), 36–40.

Stenroth, L., Peltonen, J., Cronin, N.J., Sipilä, S. & Finni, T. (2012) Age-related differences in Achilles tendon properties and triceps surae muscle architecture *in vivo*. *Journal of Applied Physiology*, **113** (**10**), 1537–1544.

CHAPTER 8

Medical Care at Major Sporting Events

Mike Loosemore[1,2]

[1]Sports Physician, English Institute of Sport, London, UK
[2]The Institute of Sport, Exercise and Health, University College London, London, UK

OVERVIEW

In this chapter, we describe the provision of medical care at major sporting events. After studying this chapter, the reader will know:

- To gain as much medical information on the team before leaving
- To plan travel to be as quick and comfortable as possible and consider effects of jet lag
- To plan for conditions in the country you are travelling to
- The role of anti-doping education for the whole team
- To prepare for emergencies

Introduction

This chapter is written assuming that a team is being taken to a major event, an Olympic or Commonwealth games, however, the advice can also be applicable to smaller events.

At a major event, particularly a multisport event, an up-to-date medical record should be obtained not only from every athlete that will be travelling to the event but also the support staff. It is key to know of any chronic medical issues that may require interventions when abroad. It is also prudent to obtain an up-to-date list of medications the athletes are taking and to ensure that none of the medication is on the WADA banned list. If the medication is on the banned list and the athlete requires it for medical reasons, then it is important that an up-to-date therapeutic use exemption (TUE) form is completed to avoid the risk of an accidental positive-doping test.

It is very useful for the team doctor to meet the athletes and support staff before the games, this allows confidence to build so that in a situation of pressurised games the medical team is not a new and unfamiliar face. The same is true of the medical team, who may never have worked together before. Meetings before the games can help relationships during the games so that the medical team can run with fewer problems.

The first thing to do is to ascertain the location of the competition, so that the correct arrangements can be made. A reconnaissance

ABC of Sports and Exercise Medicine, Fourth Edition.
Edited by Gregory P. Whyte, Mike Loosemore and Clyde Williams.
© 2015 John Wiley & Sons, Ltd. Published 2015 by John Wiley & Sons, Ltd.

visit to the location is invaluable if this is possible. A reconnaissance visit will give you the opportunity to assess local conditions at first hand and also make personal contact with staff at the organising committee and local hospitals: this will also allow you to assess the standard of the hospital and its facilities.

Before travelling
Immunisations

It is always wise to get up-to-date advice on immunisations as this advice can change with local conditions. Immunisations often have to be given well in advance of travel, as some immunisations can make the athlete unwell or cause local soreness at the injection site, for example, tetanus immunisation often causes local muscle pain for several days following immunisation. So the immunisation schedule will need to be discussed with the coach to avoid loss-of-training time in the build up to competition (also see Chapter 10 on infections).

Malaria

Malaria is a parasitic infection spread by the female Anopheles mosquitoes that are infected by *Plasmodium* parasites. The female Anopheles mosquito usually bites at dusk and at night. If you are travelling to or through a malarial region, advice should be sort as anti-malarial medication may not be required especially if the event is confined to the city, and the opposite is true if the event is in the country side within a malarial region. The resistance of local malaria strains can also change, so advice should be obtained on the correct anti-malarial medication for the specific area to which you are travelling. Even when travelling to an area with no malaria, if the journey requires the athlete or the team to stop in a malarial region, then anti-malarial medication may be required.

In addition to anti-malarial medication, there are other ways to reduce the risk of mosquito bites especially overnight, sleeping under mosquito nets and wearing long-sleeved clothing puts a physical barrier between the traveller and the mosquito that will help to prevent bites. DEET (N,N-Diethyl-metatoluamide) is a very effective insect repellent and occasionally this can cause skin irritation so a small patch of skin should be tested before use, there are various other methods available to repel mosquitoes, for example, electronic devices and slow burning coils.

Dengue fever

Dengue fever is another potentially lethal disease spread by mosquitoes. This viral haemorrhagic fever is rapidly spreading around the world, unlike the mosquitoes that spread malaria, the dengue fever mosquitoes live in very small pools of water in urban areas. At time of writing there is no medical prophylaxis that can be taken and there is no vaccine. Unlike the haemophilus mosquito, the dengue fever mosquito tends to bite during the day, so athletes rely on insect repellants such as Deet and long-sleeved tops and trousers as a physical barrier; however, this type of clothing may be implacable when training and competing. Dengue fever presents with high temperature and severe muscle pains, the patient should be transferred to hospital as soon as possible as the only treatment is supportive.

Altitude

If the event is being held above 500 m, then some adaption to altitude may be required. Adaption to altitude is very variable and some people take longer than others and some will always struggle with altitude. Preparation for altitude can be helped by sleeping in a low-oxygen tension tent replicating the low-oxygen tension of altitude. Training can continue as normal (sleep at high altitude and at low altitude).

Travelling
Mode of transport

Flying. Direct flights are preferable to flights with one or more stops, as the journey time is shorter and less stressful. Many teams if they can afford it will fly business class, especially for longer flights and also if the team contains particularly tall athletes, for example, basketball.

Travel sickness. Being able to access sub-lingual anti-nausea tablets is prudent for all journeys.

Jet lag

Jet lag describes the symptoms of trying to live at a different time zone from which your bodies' circadian rhythm is operating. Jet lag can give symptoms of extreme tiredness, nausea and headaches. The circadian rhythm is regulated by the hypothalamus, and it takes time for the production of chemicals to change to the new environment. Two of the main drivers that signal to the hypothalamus to regulate the normal circadian rhythm are day light and insulin levels. To help the body adapt to a new time zone, it is important to live at the new time zone as quickly as possible, especially exposure to sunlight and eating meals at the correct time for the new time zone. Most people find travelling from West to East more difficult, this is because you need to go to sleep when your body physiologically is still in the middle of the day, and you have to get up when the body is trying to put you in a deep sleep. To help athletes sleep in these circumstances, a short-acting sleeping tablet or a Melatonin-containing medication can be used. This may or may not speed up the adaption process, but it will stop the athlete becoming exhausted during the adaption process. As a general rule, it takes about 1 day to adapt to each hour of time difference.

At the event
Food

Differences in food will often result in diarrhoea for a couple of days on most trips. In areas where food hygiene may be poor and the tap water is not of a high enough quality to drink, gut infections can be more serious. Hand washing is the most effective way to prevent travellers' diarrhoea, and soap and warm water are best but often this is not readily available so athletes should be encouraged to use an anti-bacterial hand rub just before they eat, for example, alcohol gel. Other prophylactic methods include the use of probiotics and the use of prophylactic antibiotics. If the athlete gets diarrhoea, fluids should be replaced with an electrolyte containing sports rehydration drink. Commercial rehydration drinks work well and are often more palatable that the clinical rehydration preparations. If the athlete is competing or if the diarrhoea has been going on for 48 hours, then medication to reduce the amount of diarrhoea can be introduced, for example, Loperamide. If the athlete has a temperature over 38 °C, blood in the stool or cramping abdominal pains, then a bacterial infection should be suspected. Ideally a stool sample should be sent to establish the nature of the infection and sensitivities of the bacteria, this is however not always possible. In this situation, the antibiotic most likely to be effective should be used. In non-athletes this would be Ciprofloxacin; however, there is some evidence that this antibiotic may lead to tendon changes so it should be avoided in athletes. Instead, alternative can be used, for example, Erythromycin or Rifaximin.

Weather

The weather conditions at the event should be prepared for before travel. For example, the need for rehydration, avoiding sun burn and the symptoms of heat stroke to look out for in yourself and others in hot conditions could be taught before leaving. Extreme cold likewise requires careful preparation and training.

Wild life

Dogs. In areas where rabies is endemic and there are wild dogs roaming around it may well be worth considering a rabies vaccine before leaving. If a member of the team is bitten by a wild dog the possibility of rabies must be considered.

Rats. Sports taking place in water are at risk of contracting Weil's disease from rats' urine. In many parts of the world, Weil's disease is endemic and a high level of suspicion for Weil's disease should be maintained for flu-like illness in athletes taking part in these sports. Treatment with oral penicillin should be commenced as soon as possible.

Snakes. Snake bites are uncommon but if bitten try to kill the snake and bring to the hospital so that it can be identified and the correct anti-venom be administered.

Athlete village

On arrival at the athlete village, a medical room should be established that is private and has an examination couch, the team need to know how to contact the doctor and the location of the medical room. The medical provision in the athlete's village should be investigated, at a big games there will be a polyclinic that may have various imaging modalities from X-ray to MRI. A polyclinic will also often provide a dental service and an optician as well as other specialists who are available to treat all athletes at the games. There will also be a pharmacy with a formulary, this is often available before leaving home and is helpful in knowing which medications to bring with you to the event. It is also worth visiting the local hospitals that have been allocated for use at games time, so that you know how to locate the hospital in the case of emergency.

Covering venues

Venues where athletes are competing will have some degree of medical cover. There will be a medical room with various levels of equipment, some of which may work, and various levels of staff, some of which may work. If the team doctor feels this cover is inadequate, this should be pointed out to the games organisers and may mean that you have to bring your own kit to cover the event when your team is competing. It is crucial to know the rules for the sport you are covering, as this may be a sport you are not familiar with, especially the field of play rules. While entering the field of play to attend an injured rugby player with the game still going on is acceptable, stepping on the judo mat will get the athlete disqualified.

Equipment

If there is no polyclinic, then the team doctor must bring their own equipment. Basic equipment for travel abroad would be stethoscope, sphygmomanometer, thermometer, ophthalmoscope/otoscope, pen torch, urine-testing sticks, note book and pencil. An ultrasound machine may be very useful, but similar to any other item of equipment you need to know how to use it.

Medicines. Most medical problems encountered will be the everyday common minor illnesses, colds, coughs, diarrhoea/constipation rashes and so on, so the medication taken reflects this. If there is no pharmacy, then the team doctor needs to carry a selection of medications they may require. The following is a basic list of medications to take when travelling abroad: pain killers: Paracetamol, Codeine; non-steroidal anti-inflammatory drugs: Ibuprofen, Celebrex; antibiotics: Penicillin V (for iv use), Amoxicillin, Erythromycin, Doxycycline; eyes: chloramphenicol eye ointment; ears: Locorten vioform; gut: Loperamide, Senna, Buccastem; topical: NSAID, Canesten HC; and GTN spray. Check that all the medications packed are not on the banned list before you leave, this removes any anxiety during competition that a drug on the banned list will be accidently administered.

Language

Speaking the local language is very helpful.

Media training

The medical team do not often have to appear in front of the media during an event, but if they do it is usually bad news, a terrible injury or illness, or a positive dope test. It is therefore a good idea to get some media training so that a bad situation is not made worse.

Contingency planning. With large groups travelling and living together, infectious diseases can spread quickly through the team affecting their performance, provision for an isolation room should be made to prevent spread. Plans on how to repatriate patients home if they are very ill should be made.

Expecting the unexpected

Rare medical emergencies do occur, such as severe mental illness, meningitis, ruptured kidney and even lightning strike.

Choosing a medical team. If you have the luxury of having a large medical team, it is helpful as they have a range of skills and are familiar with different sports.

Doping. A positive-doping result will have major repercussions not only on the athlete but also for the reputation of the team. Education of the team is key to avoiding an accidental positive dope test. National anti-doping organisations will often have ready-made education programmes for athletes. All athletes should be constantly reminded not to take any medication, including that prescribed by a doctor, the team manager or their mother, without checking if it is on the banned list by contacting the team doctor or checking online. www.globaldro.com is very useful. On arrival at the accommodation, the team doctor will go through each individual's medication and supplements even to the extent of examining the packaging to try to ensure that the athlete does not get an accidental positive-doping result by taking a medication or supplement that contains a banned substance. Whereabouts is the system where the anti-doping authorities are informed by the team where athletes are going to be during the games so that random doping tests can be carried out. The whereabouts procedure requires a great deal of administrative time and is best left to the team manager as mistakes can lead to missed tests that can result in athletes being banned. TUE forms need to be submitted to the games organisers usually 4–6 weeks before the event. Emergency TUEs required at the games will need to be submitted to the games anti-doping committee.

Summary

Prepare well by gaining as much information as possible on the team travelling and the local conditions at the destination. Reduce travel stress by taking into account jet lag and by choosing the most comfortable mode of travel. On arrival, make local contacts so that there is a pathway to treat members of the team if you do not have the appropriate resources. Expect the unexpected and ensure that pathways of communication in the case of emergency are clear before you travel. Enjoy the event!

Further reading

Devitt, B.M. & McCarthy, C. (2010) 'I am in blood Stepp'd in so far …': ethical dilemmas and the sports team doctor. *British Journal of Sports Medicine*, **44** (3), 175–178. doi:10.1136/bjsm.2009.068056.

Tillett, E. & Loosemore, M. (2009) Setting standards for the prevention and management of travellers' diarrhoea in elite athletes: an audit of one team during the Youth Commonwealth Games in India. *British Journal of Sports Medicine*, **43** (13), 1045–1048. doi:10.1136/bjsm.2009.063396. Epub 2009 Oct 25.

CHAPTER 9

Pulmonary Dysfunction in Athletes

John Dickinson[1] and James Hull[2]

[1]University of Kent, Chatham Maritime, UK
[2]The Royal Brompton Hospital, Sydney Street, London, UK

OVERVIEW

- Exercise-induced bronchoconstriction (EIB) is the most prevalent chronic medical condition in elite athletes
- Athletes are at risk of EIB if their sport involves sustained high minute ventilation or takes place in a provocative environment (e.g. dry air or pollution)
- Several conditions mimic EIB (e.g. 'dysfunctional breathing' or upper airway dysfunction), and therefore a secure diagnosis is dependent on objective testing (i.e. bronchoprovocation testing)
- Indirect airway challenge tests are the best means to diagnose EIB in athletes
- Treatment of EIB should involve both pharmacological and non-pharmacological strategies.

Introduction

Pulmonary physiology in athletes

The pulmonary system adapts during exercise in order to maintain performance and minimise airway resistance, despite a significant increase in airflow. This process involves a complex and synchronous interaction between respiratory skeletal muscles and bronchial smooth muscle, acting to facilitate the rise in tidal volume while minimising elastic work performed by the respiratory muscles. Thus, in healthy individuals, the demands placed on the respiratory system during exercise do not stress the limits of capacity within the system.

It is often expected that athletes will have supra-normal resting lung physiology values. However, studies reveal that lung volumes generally reflect genetic influences and body size characteristics of an individual. Indeed, there is limited evidence to suggest that exercise training alters the structural parameters of the respiratory system. This acknowledged lung volume is related to aerobic capacity; therefore, in a group of athletes for whom aerobic capacity is an important component of success (e.g. endurance athletes), average lung volumes will tend to be higher than in the general population.

ABC of Sports and Exercise Medicine, Fourth Edition.
Edited by Gregory P. Whyte, Mike Loosemore and Clyde Williams.

The normal response of the airways to intense physical activity is to dilate. This bronchial dilation is characterised physiologically by an increase in airflow measures, for example, forced expiratory volume in 1 s (FEV_1). This dilatation is evident for up to an hour following exercise cessation.

Pulmonary symptoms in athletes

Pulmonary symptoms are common in athletes of all abilities. Indeed in a questionnaire study of 700 athletes, nearly a quarter reported the presence of regular, troublesome respiratory symptoms.

A key problem for the clinician encountering an athlete with pulmonary symptoms is differentiating between those indicating underlying cardiorespiratory pathology from symptoms or 'sensations' that fall within a spectrum of what could be considered 'physiologically normal' or appropriate in the setting of intense exercise. To this end, research reveals that respiratory symptoms in athletes are often non-specific and often described with nociceptive terminology; for example, 'I feel that my breathing is rapid' or 'I feel that I am breathing more'. This might explain, at least in part, the poor relation between the presence of 'asthma-type' symptoms (e.g. cough and chest discomfort) and objective evidence of airways disease in athletes (see differential diagnosis for EIB later).

The most frequently encountered pulmonary condition in athletes is airways disease. Indeed EIB is the most common chronic medical condition in elite athletes and is highly prevalent in athletes of all abilities (Table 9.1). This chapter therefore focuses on

Table 9.1 Prevalence of EIB in sport

Sport	Prevalence (%)	Winter sport	Sustained high minute ventilation	Presence of air pollution
Badminton	9			
Amateur boxing	12			
Athletics	16		X	
Soccer	29	X	X	
Rowing	31		X	
Rugby	35	X	X	
Cycling	40		X	X
Swimming	44		X	X
Biathlon	45	X	X	

providing a pragmatic overview of the assessment and management of suspected EIB.

Exercise-induced bronchoconstriction

The term EIB is used to describe transient and reversible narrowing of the airways that occurs in association with exercise. It is often used interchangeably with the term exercise-induced asthma (EIA); however, EIB is favoured given that exercise triggers bronchoconstriction, but does not induce the clinical syndrome of asthma.

The prevalence of EIB in a cohort of athletes varies dependent on sport and tends to be highest in cohorts of athletes partaking in sports that have high aerobic demands and/or take place in provocative or potentially noxious environments (e.g. cold climate, chlorinated swimming pool) (Table 9.1). Despite this, EIB is also prevalent in recreational gym users and non-elite athletic groups partaking in popular field-based sports (e.g. soccer).

Diagnosis of EIB

The presentation of EIB in an athlete is often characterised by a broad spectrum of symptoms including wheeze, cough, chest tightness, dyspnoea and excess mucus production. Studies have revealed, however, that in athletes these symptoms are non-specific and as such actually provide no diagnostic precision in the diagnosis of EIB. It is therefore recommended that a diagnosis of EIB in an athlete should not be based on symptoms alone. Accordingly, in order to establish a secure diagnosis, it is recommended that an athlete has objective testing to demonstrate reversible airflow obstruction. This can be achieved by evaluating response either to bronchodilator medication or to exercise or bronchoprovocation testing (Figure 9.1). The International Olympic Committee – Medical Commission recommend indirect airway challenge testing as the gold standard means to establish a diagnosis of EIB in a competitive athlete.

Bronchodilator challenge

Bronchodilator challenges are favoured in athletes with evidence of airflow obstruction at rest. A rise in FEV_1 of $\geq 12\%$ and 200 ml or more 10 min after inhaling a short-acting β_2 agonist (400 µg of inhaled Salbutamol) provides evidence of reversible airflow obstruction (Figure 9.2).

The vast majority of athletes with respiratory symptoms will have resting FEV_1 values within the normal range (> 80% of their predicted value). In these individuals, an indirect airway challenge is the most appropriate means of establishing a diagnosis.

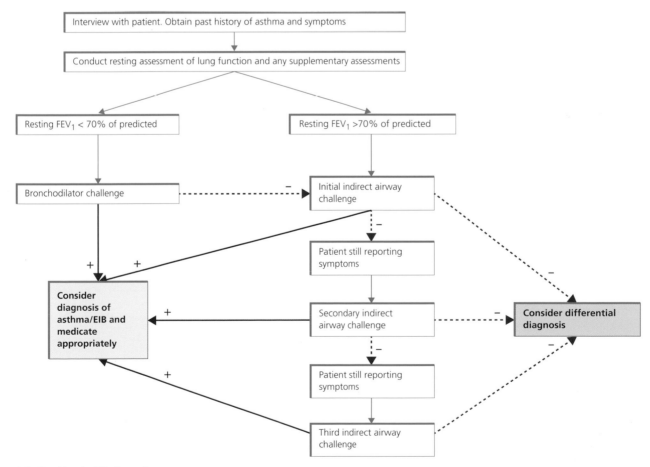

Figure 9.1 Algorithm for EIB diagnosis

Dialog box: How to measure a maximal flow volume loop

• Use a spirometer that meets American Thoracic Society/European Respiratory Society standards.

• Instruct the athlete to take several relaxed breathes prior to instructing them to inhale until they reach total lung capacity.

• Once the athlete reaches total lung capacity they should immediately expire should be as hard and as fast as possible until they can't breathe anymore air out (reached residual volume).

• From residual volume the athlete should immediately inspire air as fast as possible until they reach total lung capacity. The measurement of the maximal flow-volume loop is now complete.

• For the assessment of resting lung function three flow loops should be measured. The best FEV_1, from the three flow loops can be recorded. All other flow-volume measures should be taken from the flow-volume loop with the best combined FEV_1 and FVC as long as the variance between the three flow loops is no greater than 5%.

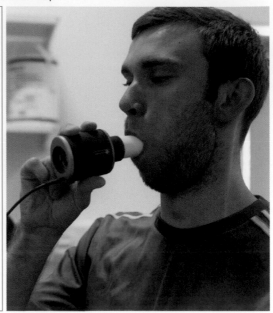

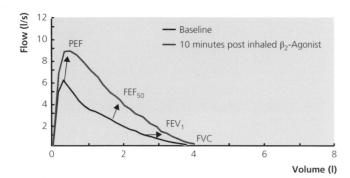

Figure 9.2 Positive bronchodilator challenge. This is an example of a bronchodilator challenge where the FEV_1 increases >12% following inhaled β_2-agonist. Note that the FVC does not change, but the flow rate throughout the maximal expiratory effort improves and the shape of the loop from PEF to FVC changes from a concave shape towards a liner shape

Indirect airway challenges

Indirect airway challenges (e.g. exercise challenge, eucapnic voluntary hyperpnoea (EVH) and mannitol challenge) are thought to be the most sensitive challenges to diagnose EIB in athletes (Table 9.2).

They are termed 'indirect' challenges because a positive response is dependent on activation of a cascade in the airways, that is, dependent on the release of mediators that then cause airway smooth muscle contraction. It is argued that this simulates the real-life situation that occurs when an athlete exercises and is thus thought to be more pertinent in athletes than a direct bronchoprovocation challenge (e.g. Methacholine). Figure 9.3 demonstrates the expected flow–volume response to an indirect airway challenge from an athlete with EIB.

Exercise challenge

Exercise challenge testing is a type of indirect airway challenge for EIB. It is recommended that the exercise challenge is undertaken

Table 9.2 Classification of EIB severity based on %MVV during EVH challenge

FEV_1 fall to following EVH challenge	Minute ventilation <60% MVV	Minute ventilation >60% MVV
<10%	Normal[a]	Normal
10–20%	Moderate	Mild
20–30%	Moderate	Moderate
>30%	Severe	Severe

[a]Interpretation of FEV_1 fall <10% from baseline must be taken with caution if minute ventilation achieved during the EVH challenge is <60% MVV. If athlete continues to present with symptoms, consider alternative indirect airway challenge to confirm diagnosis.

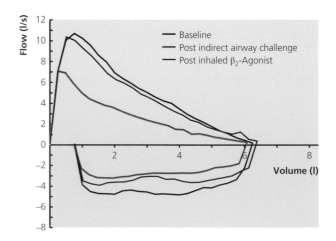

Figure 9.3 Positive indirect airway challenge. This is an example of the maximal flow–volume loops you may see from a positive indirect airway challenge. Note that the FVC does not change post-challenge, but the flow rate is reduced and the shape of the expiratory curve becomes concave indicating bronchoconstriction. Following inhalation of short acting β_2-agonist, the bronchoconstriction is reversed and lung function returns to that seen at baseline

in a sport-specific setting, that is, performed in the environment in which an athlete's symptoms are commonly reported (e.g. swimmer undergoes exercise challenge in the pool).

The exercise challenge involves measuring maximal flow–volume loops at rest and following exercise. The exercise challenge should incorporate a 2-min warm-up directly followed by approximately 8 min of exercise that sustains a heart rate >80% of predicted heart rate max. Following the exercise, duplicate flow–volume loops should be taken at regular time points up to 30 min post-exercise. The greatest fall in FEV_1 is usually seen between 3 and 10 min post-exercise challenge. To capture the maximum fall in FEV_1, measurements of maximal flow–volume are typically recorded 3, 5, 7, 10 and 15 min post-exercise. A test is regarded as positive if FEV_1 falls 10% or more from rest at two consecutive time points during the post-exercise spirometry manoeuvres.

Eucapnic voluntary hyperpnoea challenge

The EVH challenge (Figure 9.4) is regarded as the most sensitive indirect airway challenge to diagnose EIB. As such, it is often referred to as the 'gold-standard', however, work is ongoing to establish if the test is too sensitive and 'detects' EIB in athletes who are otherwise asymptomatic and have no deleterious performance or health implications from their 'EIB'.

Maximal flow–volume loops are measured in a similar way to the exercise challenge at rest and following the EVH challenge. During the EVH challenge, the athlete is required to breathe at 85% of their maximum voluntary ventilation (MVV) rate ($30 \times FEV_1$) for 6 min. Achieving 85% MVV is only made possible by the participant inhaling gas from a compressed gas cylinder that contains 5% CO_2, 21% O_2 and 74% N_2, to stop the athlete succumbing to hypocapnoea.

A positive test is regarded as a fall in FEV_1 of 10% or greater from rest at two consecutive time points post-EVH challenge. The interpretation of the test should consider the degree of fall in FEV_1 and the ventilation achieved (Table 9.2).

Mannitol challenge

The mannitol challenge test (Aridol, Pharmaxis Ltd, Australia) has a similar sensitivity and specificity to an EVH challenge in summer

athletes. However, in winter athletes, it is thought to have a reduced sensitivity in the diagnosis of EIB when compared with an EVH challenge. A mannitol challenge may be most appropriate for the initial testing of sub-elite athletes. It may also be appropriate for athletes who are negative to an EVH challenge but report increased symptoms related to exercise in atopic environments (e.g. pollen). The protocol for mannitol testing is described in Figure 9.5.

Supportive and follow-up assessments

A positive response to an indirect airway challenge provides objective support for a diagnosis of EIB. However, it may be beneficial to carry out additional assessments to optimise ongoing care for an athlete.

Ancillary tests may be used to provide information regarding active airway inflammation (e.g. exhaled nitric oxide) and may provide a monitoring tool to indicate how inhaled therapy should be adjusted. Skin prick testing to common aeroallergens can also be used to identify relevant atopic triggers.

Following the diagnosis of EIB and initiation of appropriate therapy (discussed in the following section), it may be appropriate to repeat an indirect airway challenge in a competitive athlete while on medication. Results from this follow-up assessment will inform and refine future treatment and ensure optimal protection against EIB.

Screening for EIB

The poor relationship between symptoms and objective diagnosis of EIB has led some to recommend screening squads of athletes for EIB using indirect airway challenges. The benefit of this approach was highlighted when the author screened the British Olympic Squad in 2004. It was subsequently revealed that many athletes were competing with an incorrect diagnosis of EIB. Moreover, the assessment process revealed that many athletes do not recognise and/or report exercise respiratory symptoms and therefore train and compete with uncontrolled EIB. Screening for EIB, using an indirect airway challenge, removes diagnostic uncertainty and can ensure optimal care for an athlete.

Treatment for EIB

Both pharmacological and non-pharmacological interventions should be considered in the treatment of airways disease in athletes (see Table 9.3).

Non-pharmacological

Performing a high-intensity, interval warm-up (i.e. bursts of high-intensity exercise interspersed with periods of low-intensity exercise) takes advantage of a refractory period (i.e. time when EIB will not recur if an athlete has exercised) in up to half of athletes and should be encouraged. Dietary interventions and strategies to humidify inspired air (e.g. face muffle) may also prove beneficial (see American Thoracic Society (ATS) recommendations from reading list).

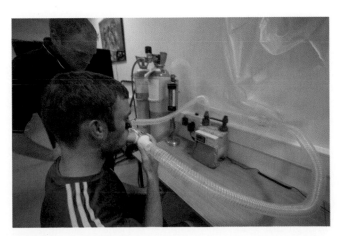

Figure 9.4 EVH challenge

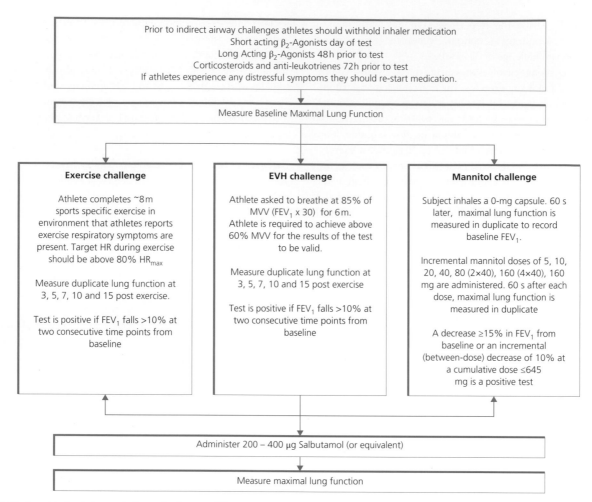

Prior to indirect airway challenges athletes should withhold inhaler medication
Short acting β_2-Agonists day of test
Long Acting β_2-Agonists 48h prior to test
Corticosteroids and anti-leukotrienes 72h prior to test
If athletes experience any distressful symptoms they should re-start medication.

Measure Baseline Maximal Lung Function

Exercise challenge

Athlete completes ~8m sports specific exercise in environment that athletes reports exercise respiratory symptoms are present. Target HR during exercise should be above 80% HR_{max}

Measure duplicate lung function at 3, 5, 7, 10 and 15 post exercise.

Test is positive if FEV_1 falls >10% at two consecutive time points from baseline

EVH challenge

Athlete asked to breathe at 85% of MVV (FEV_1 x 30) for 6m. Athlete is required to achieve above 60% MVV for the results of the test to be valid.

Measure duplicate lung function at 3, 5, 7, 10 and 15 post exercise

Test is positive if FEV_1 falls >10% at two consecutive time points from baseline

Mannitol challenge

Subject inhales a 0-mg capsule. 60 s later, maximal lung function is measured in duplicate to record baseline FEV_1.

Incremental mannitol doses of 5, 10, 20, 40, 80 (2×40), 160 (4×40), 160 mg are administered. 60 s after each dose, maximal lung function is measured in duplicate

A decrease ≥15% in FEV_1 from baseline or an incremental (between-dose) decrease of 10% at a cumulative dose ≤645 mg is a positive test

Administer 200 – 400 µg Salbutamol (or equivalent)

Measure maximal lung function

Figure 9.5 Choice of indirect airway challenge to diagnose EIB

Table 9.3 Management strategies for EIB

Pharmacological	Non-pharmacological
Inhaled short-acting β_2-agonists (e.g. salbutamol, terbutaline)	High-intensity warm-up
Inhaled long-acting β_2-agonists (e.g. salmeterol, formoterol)	Avoidance of triggers
Inhaled corticosteriods (e.g. beclomethasone, fluticasone dipropinate)	Wear mask covering nose and mouth in cold and dry environments
Cromolyn compounds (e.g. sodium cromoglycate)	Diet high in Omega-3 fatty acids (3 g of eicosapentaenoic acid and 2 g of docohexaenoic acid) daily
Leukotriene modifiers (e.g. montelukast)	

Pharmacological

Inhaled short-acting β-2 agonists form the mainstay of treatment and when administered 15 min prior to exercise are usually effective in negating EIB. Further treatment should be guided by the frequency of requirement of β-2 agonist therapy and presence of additional symptoms. It is recommended that athletes who have asthma symptoms that occur outside the setting of exercise or who frequently use β-2 agonist medication (i.e. more than three times per week) should be treated with anti-inflammatory agent; for example, regular inhaled corticosteroid or an oral leukotriene antagonist. The optimum anti-inflammatory treatment for EIB in athletes is not established; however, guidelines from the European and American Thoracic Societies (see further reading) provide up-to-date guidance and indicate suitable regimes. It is vitally important that an athlete's inhaler technique is checked and optimised.

Very few inhaled asthma medications remain prohibited for use in therapeutic quantities by the World Anti-Doping Agency. Athletes should however be able to provide clinical evidence to support their requirement to take inhaled asthma medication (i.e. be able to provide physician proof of a clinical assessment). The list of prohibited substances is frequently updated, and therefore it is advisable to view www.globaldro.org or consult with the relevant national anti-doping agency. In the context of an exacerbation in asthma, oral corticosteroid remains prohibited in competition and therefore a therapeutic use exemption is required (see Chapter 23).

Differential diagnosis for EIB

Although EIB is the most common respiratory condition diagnosed in athletes, it is not uncommon to encounter athletes who

Table 9.4 Differences between EIB and EILO

EIB	EILO
Symptoms occur 5–10 min after exercise	Symptoms occur during exercise and resolve within 5 min of stopping exercise
Wheeze on expiration	Wheeze on inspiration
Fall in FEV_1 following indirect airway challenge	No fall in FEV_1 following indirect airway challenge
Sound is primarily from the chest	Sound originates in the neck
EIA responds to inhaled β_2-agonists treatment	No response to inhaled β_2-agonists treatment

report troublesome exercise-associated respiratory symptoms in the absence of EIB. The differential diagnosis for EIB is broad and includes cardiac disease (see Chapter 10). However, it is our experience that in the absence of evidence of clinical or investigation findings that indicate other cardiorespiratory disease, an athlete's exertional dyspnoea often arises secondary to 'dysfunctional breathing'.

Several entities can account for 'dysfunctional breathing', including an exercise-associated breathing pattern disorder or upper airway dysfunction. A breathing pattern disorder may arise as the results of inappropriate activation of accessory muscles (e.g. deltoids and pectorals) to initiate inspiratory manoeuvres during exercise.

It is also now recognised that in a significant proportion of young/adolescent athletes, symptoms attributed to EIB may actually arise from an exercise associated narrowing at the level of the larynx. This condition termed exercise-induced laryngeal obstruction (EILO) is a prevalent cause for unexplained dyspnoea in athletes and has several overlapping features with EIB (see Table 9.4).

The diagnosis of dysfunctional breathing is not straightforward and requires assessment by individuals with expertise, employing clinical observation during high-intensity exercise and technology to capture chest and abdomen wall movements during and following exercise. Confirmation of EILO requires direct nasendoscopy during exercise, and it should be recognised that

there is a considerable overlap between EIB and EILO; that is, some athletes will have both conditions thus rendering them 'refractory' to EIB treatment alone.

The optimum treatment of dysfunctional breathing and EILO is yet to be established; however, breathing technique training, core stability improvement and respiratory muscle training are beneficial. Thoracic myofacial release massage may also be beneficial to improve chest compliance and relieve symptoms.

Summary

Respiratory symptoms are common in athletes of all abilities, and indeed asthma is the most prevalent chronic medication condition reported in elite athletes. Despite this, it is important to recognise that exercise-associated respiratory symptoms may not arise from bronchoconstriction but from a differential diagnosis that includes transient upper airway obstruction and/or dysfunctional breathing. A secure diagnostic assessment is therefore dependent on objective testing.

Further reading

Anderson, S. & Kippelen, P. (2012) Assessment and prevention of exercise-induced bronchoconstriction. *British Journal of Sports Medicine*, **46**, 391–396.

Dickinson, J., McConnell, A. & Whyte, G. (2011) Diagnosis of exercise-induced bronchoconstriction: eucapnic voluntary hyperpnoea challenges identify previously undiagnosed elite athletes with exercise-induced bronchoconstriction. *British Journal of Sports Medicine*, **45**, 1126–1131.

Nielsen, E., Hull, J. & Backer, V. (2013) High prevalence of exercise-induced laryngeal obstruction in athletes. *Medicine and Science in Sports and Exercise*, **45**, 2030–2035.

Parsons, J., Hallstrand, T., Mastronarde, J. *et al.* (2013) An official American Thoracic Society clinical practice guideline: exercise-induced bronchoconstriction. *American Journal of Respiratory and Critical Care Medicine*, **187** (**9**), 1016–1027.

Porsbjerg, C. & Brannan, J. (2010) Alternatives to exercise challenge for the objective assessment of exercise induced bronchospasm: eucapnic voluntary hyperpnoea and the osmotic challenge tests. *Breathe*, **7**, 53–63.

CHAPTER 10

Infections

Michael J. Martin

Royal Bournemouth Hospital, Bournemouth, UK

OVERVIEW

- Certain infections are increasingly being recognised as associated with specific sports
- We now recognise that many of these can be avoided by prior education and preparation
- Attention to hygiene plays a very important part in preventing infections particularly in contact sports
- It is no longer acceptable for athletes in contact sports suffering a blood injury to continue playing without appropriate treatment
- Doctors at sporting events need appropriate equipment and may need specific training, particularly at elite level

An increasing number of people participating in a wider variety of sports mean that many types of infection may now be associated with sport. Increasing international competition and proliferation of adventure holidays also means that unusual infections must be considered not only in elite athletes but also in holidaymakers returning from activity holidays.

Proper preparation for athletes prior to departure is essential if foreign travel will be involved. Diarrhoeal illness is common in many parts of the world and advice should include dietary advice about drinking bottled water where local water supplies may be of poor quality and avoiding salads, unpeeled fruits and ice in drinks. Vaccines should be considered, some weeks in advance of departure, depending on the destination. Advice about these is available in *The Green Book* (see later).

Skin and soft tissue infections

Viral skin infections

The two most common viral skin infections are verrucas and the Herpes simplex viruses. Verrucas caused by the human papillomavirus can be found on any skin surface and are transmitted by direct contact. Changing facility floors can act as a reservoir and plantar warts are common in swimmers. Although plantar warts can be painful as the wart is pushed inwards by pressure, most warts are painless. Early treatment with topical salicylic acid preparations daily for several weeks may be effective, but more established warts, particularly plantar warts, may need more aggressive therapy including cryotherapy with liquid nitrogen, surgical excision or laser therapy. Herpes simplex infection, when seen in wrestlers is referred to as herpes gladiatorum and in rugby players as scrumpox (Figure 10.1), is common in contact and combat sports and presents as vesicles with surrounding erythema that are often extremely painful. Rupture may follow leaving eroded ulcerated areas. Lymphadenopathy, fever and general malaise are often seen. Treatment with Aciclovir 200 mg five times daily for 5 days is indicated and exclusion of the competitor until the lesions has healed.

Fungal skin infections

Fungal skin infections with dermatophytes are common in athletes. Tinea pedis characterised by scaling or discrete lesions on the foot is common. Interdigital maceration can occur because the organism thrives in warm, moist environments. Runners and walkers are most at risk. Tinea corporis is usually found as scaly erythematous plaques, a form of which, tinea corporis gladiatorum, is well recognised among wrestlers. Transmission is by close personal contact, although mats and equipment may sometimes be implicated. Pityriasis versicolor is caused by Malassezia group of yeasts, members of the normal skin flora, characteristically causing a rash, usually on the trunk, of oval or irregular spots of hypo- or hyperpigmentation that may coalesce. Various topical imidazole antifungal creams are available for dermatophytes (e.g. clotrimazole, ketoconazole and miconazole) as well as selenium sulphide or ketoconazole shampoo for pityriasis versicolor.

Bacterial skin infections
Impetigo

Impetigo is a usually a mild localised skin infection. It was classically caused by *Streptococcus pyogenes* (Group A streptococci), though now *Staphylococcus aureus* is by far the most common cause. It is common where skin abrasions are found and so occurs in a variety of sports and is more common in hot humid weather.

ABC of Sports and Exercise Medicine, Fourth Edition.
Edited by Gregory P. Whyte, Mike Loosemore and Clyde Williams.

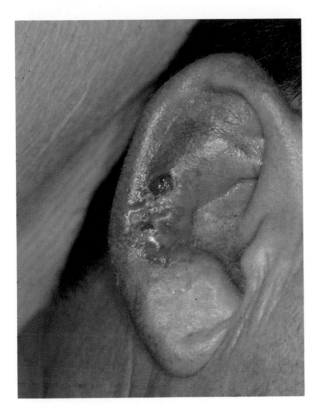

Figure 10.1 Herpes simplex – 'scrumpox'

It begins as small vesicles that become pustules before rupturing and crusting over to form characteristic golden yellow crusts. It can be intensely pruritic, and scratching can lead to further spread. Mild cases may respond to cleaning with antiseptic and allowing the lesion to dry up. Topical Mupirocin ointment t.d.s. (three times daily) for 5 days is effective, although more serious infections may require oral Flucloxacillin 250 mg q.d.s. (four times daily) or erythromycin 250 mg q.d.s. for 5 days. Exclusion of the competitor until healing has occurred is necessary, and it is important to be vigilant as team mates may also develop lesions.

Staphylococcus aureus and the Panton–Valentine leucocidin toxin

Panton–Valentine leucocidin (PVL) is a toxin that is produced by around 2% of strains of *S. aureus*. It can be found in both meticillin-sensitive (MSSA) and meticillin-resistant (MRSA) strains. PVL producing *S. aureus* (PVL-SA) can cause recurrent skin and soft tissue infections (SSTIs) in otherwise fit young people and occasionally a life-threatening necrotising pneumonia particularly in the setting of post-influenza respiratory infections. As the name suggests, the toxin causes destruction of white blood cells including neutrophils and macrophages, allowing spread of infection and tissue destruction. Common infections with this organism include recurrent furuncles (boils), carbuncles, folliculitis and cellulitis. Spread of this organism can occur among crowded communities where close contact can occur such as gymnasia, contact sports, prisons and military establishments. Wherever there is compromised skin integrity coupled with close contact and the

possibility of the use of shared equipment including towels, then the risk of spread of PVL-SA is increased. Outbreaks have been associated with combat sports that predispose to skin breaks including wrestling, kick boxing and cage fighting as well as team sports such as rugby. A specimen from the lesion and also from the anterior nares (to look for *S. aureus* carriage) should be sent for culture in patients with necrotising SSTIs, recurrent abscesses and boils and wherever there is a suggestion of spread, such as two or more cases in a sports team. It is important to indicate on the request that PVL screening is required as this test is not routinely performed in diagnostic laboratories unless specifically requested. Antibiotics used to treat minor skin infections include Flucloxacillin 500 mg qds for 5 days. Erythromycin 500 mg qds or Clarithromycin 500 mg bd (twice daily) can be used in penicillin-allergic patients. In more serious and/or recurrent infections, Clindamycin 450 mg qds is preferred. Clindamycin works on the bacterial ribosome to stop protein synthesis, and hence toxin production. Should it be suspected or confirmed that the organism is a MRSA, Clindamycin may still be effective although combination therapy with Rifampicin 300 mg bd plus doxycycline 100 mg bd may be an alternative. Culture and sensitivity testing are essential to ensure appropriate therapy. Risk of spread to others can be reduced by sensible hygiene precautions such as covering infected lesions with a dressing, regular hand washing with pump action liquid soap (avoid the use of bars of soap – they can later be used by others who may pick up the infection), use of individual towels and facecloths and laundering these daily in a hot wash. Failure to control spread may require more extensive measures including daily washing of bed linen and disinfection of the environment. Decolonisation of persistent carriers may be necessary and is best achieved by a combination of daily antiseptic bath washes combined with nasal mupirocin ointment (Box 10.1)

Box 10.1 Decolonisation procedure for PVL-SA

General

- Sheets/towels/facecloths changed daily and washed in a hot wash
- Regular vacuuming and dusting, especially bedrooms
- Do not share toiletries
- Clean sink/bath with disposable cloth and detergent

Body wash with Chlorhexidine 4% body wash OR Triclosan 2%

- Apply daily to moistened skin for 5 days and leave for at least 1 min. Rinse thoroughly
- Use also as a shampoo on days 1, 3 and 5
- Do NOT apply to dry skin
- Pay particular attention to armpits, groins, under breasts, hands and buttocks

Mupirocin (Bactroban nasal) ointment (three times daily for 5 days)

- Apply a matchstick head-sized amount on a cotton wool bud to the inside of each nostril. Press the sides of the nose together and massage gently to spread the ointment

Upper respiratory tract infections

Upper respiratory tract infections are common not only in athletes but throughout the whole population and may affect the athlete's performance. These are readily spread, particularly by direct contact, and careful attention to hand hygiene may reduce the risk of spread. There is little harm in exercising with mild coryzal symptoms, although exercise should be avoided if the athlete is febrile, has myalgia, lethargy or joint pains or has a resting tachycardia. Infectious mononucleosis (glandular fever) can occasionally result in prolonged periods of lethargy. During convalescence, activity should be re-introduced gradually in accordance with the tolerance of the individual. Splenomegaly is common in glandular fever, and there are reported cases of splenic rupture following a premature return to contact sport.

Blood-borne viruses

Athletes may be at risk of contracting Hepatitis B and C and the Human Immunodeficiency Virus (HIV) by participating in sports involving close contact, although there have not been any documented cases of HIV transmission as a result of sporting activities to date. The viruses may be transmitted by contact with blood and body fluids. Athletes are more likely to be exposed to these viruses in activities away from the sports field, but a number of sensible hygiene practices when dealing with bleeding injuries can minimise the risk of transmission. Hygienic changing facilities should be available and good practice should be encouraged, for example, not sharing towels and razors. Protective equipment should be used where appropriate, such as mouth guards. Equipment contaminated with blood should be removed from the field of play and cleaned using, for example, a solution of 1 part household bleach to 10 parts water. Bleeding injuries should be treated promptly (Box 10.2). The athlete should leave the field of play. Gloves should be worn by the attendants. Thorough cleaning with an antiseptic should be performed and clothing should be changed if blood stained. Athletes should be educated and encouraged to report such injuries. Skin injuries should be covered with occlusive dressings until healed. Hepatitis B is the most readily spread virus, and there is a vaccine available and consideration should be given to immunising athletes at high risk or who are travelling to countries where the incidence is high.

> **Box 10.2 Action in the event of a blood injury at a sporting event**
>
> - The athlete should leave the field of play immediately
> - Gloves should be worn by the attendant
> - Thorough cleaning with antiseptic should be performed
> - Blood-stained clothing should be changed and contaminated equipment should be cleaned with dilute bleach solution
> - The injury should be covered with an occlusive dressing

> **Box 10.3 Lyme disease**
>
> - Transmitted by tick bites
> - The tick must be attached for >24 h to transmit the disease so early tick removal will prevent infection (check particularly folds of skin)
> - ECM, the classic spreading skin rash, can develop several days to several weeks after the bite
> - The rash should be treated with antibiotics. Serological testing should NOT be performed at this stage – it remains negative for several weeks after infection
> - Appropriate antibiotics include amoxicillin, doxycycline, cefuroxime axetil. Azithromycin may be used in the penicillin allergic child
> - Ten days of antibiotic therapy is adequate

Lyme disease

Lyme disease (Box 10.3) is a systemic infection caused by the spirochaete, *Borrelia burgdorferi*. It usually follows the bite of a tick of the genus *Ixodes*, commonly associated with deer. A useful rule of thumb is that Lyme is found wherever there are deer such as temperate-wooded areas in the northern hemisphere. The popularity of country-side pursuits, such as mountain biking, means that a larger number of people are putting themselves at risk. The tick feeds for several days before detaching when fully engorged, and the infection is not transmitted until the tick has been attached for at least 24 h. Therefore, it is good practice to check for ticks soon after leaving an infested area and in any event before 24 h have elapsed. Ticks particularly like the skin folds because they are warm and moist, so consider axillae, breasts, groins and popliteal fossae. It is important to note that the majority of infections are asymptomatic. Some patients will develop the characteristic rash of Erythema Chronicum Migrans (ECM), an erythematous rash (Figure 10.2) spreading outwards from the site of the bite. This usually occurs about 7 days after the bite and may be delayed until several weeks

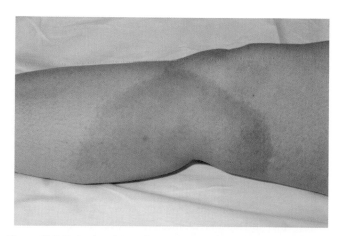

Figure 10.2 Rash of erythema chronicum migrans

later. The rash will eventually spontaneously disappear, and a few patients will go on to suffer the sequelae of chronic infection including most commonly arthritis and neurological involvement. Serological markers for the disease are not detectable for around 6 weeks after infection, so ECM should always be treated empirically with antibiotics and serological testing should not be performed. Treatment is with oral amoxicillin, cefuroxime axetil or doxycycline. Azithromycin is less effective but is an option in the penicillin allergic child. Ten days of treatment is adequate. The rash will usually take about 2 weeks to resolve.

Leptospirosis

Leptospirosis (Box 10.4) is caused by a spirochaete of the genus *Leptospira*, of which there are a number of subtypes. Although primarily a disease of tropical regions, it is found worldwide. Leptospires are excreted in the urine of many mammals, particularly that of rodents, and are found in water contaminated with such urine (fresh water lakes, streams and rivers). It can enter the skin through cuts and abrasions but can also cross intact mucous membranes. Person to person spread does not occur. Canoeists, potholers, windsurfers and swimmers may be at risk. The disease has an incubation period of 7–21 days. The infection may be asymptomatic (the majority) or may cause the abrupt onset of a flu-like illness with headache, muscle ache and vomiting. Occasional cases will then progress to the immune phase (Weil's disease), a severe illness with jaundice and hepatorenal failure. Antibiotic therapy (Penicillin) and good supportive treatment will result in complete recovery in the vast majority of cases, with death remaining rare. Athletes in contact with fresh water can be offered the following advice. Wear appropriate protective clothing. Cover cuts and scratches with a waterproof occlusive dressing. Wash or shower after water sports. Wash hands after handling animals and before eating.

Summary

Asking a patient about their leisure activities as part of history taking can help identify potential infective problems. The cornerstones to minimising risk of infection in sport, as in many areas of life, are proper preparation (including appropriate immunisation) and good hygiene (emphasising not sharing razors, bars of soap and towels). There are careers now available for doctors in the exciting field of sports medicine.

Further reading

Centers for Disease Control and Prevention, Atlanta, USA (contains topical information on all infectious diseases): www.cdc.gov.

Public Health England website (contains topical information on all infectious diseases): http://www.hpa.org.uk/.

Schlossburg, D. (ed) (2009) *Infections of Leisure*. ASM Press, Washington. ISBN 978-1-55581-484-7.

The Green Book (immunisation): https://www.gov.uk/government/collections/immunisation-against-infectious-disease-the-green-book#the-green-book.

CHAPTER 11

The Unexplained Underperformance Syndrome (Overtraining Syndrome)

Richard Budgett[1] and Yorck Olaf Schumacher[2]

[1]Medical Services, International Olympic Committee, Lausanne, Switzerland
[2]Aspetar Orthopedic and Sports Medicine Hospital, Doha, Qatar

---

OVERVIEW

In this chapter, we describe the unexplained underperformance syndrome of the athlete (overtraining syndrome). After studying this chapter, the reader will know:

- the causes
- the clinical signs
- the value of the different diagnostic tools
- the best therapeutic approach

Athletes aim to improve their performance through training. Training will initiate reconstruction and remodelling processes in their body and thereby ideally lead to an adaptation to the trained task, which subsequently results in a better performance (following the typical fatigue after training). Typically, the adaptation will occur while the athlete is fatigued during the recovery period. Sometimes, this process is amplified through very hard training interventions followed by prolonged periods of rest to increase the effect of training (so-called functional overreaching). When exhaustive training and other stressors occur simultaneously over an extended period of time together with insufficient recovery, this process is disturbed (so-called non-functional overreaching). This balance between stress and recovery is a highly individual, dynamic process and can ultimately result in long-term underperformance. These forms of unexplained underperformance syndrome (UUPS) are rather common in elite endurance athletes: 60% of all endurance runners are thought to go through periods of overreaching or overtraining during their career. The problem is not confined to Olympic athletes; 10% of collegiate swimmers in the United States are described as 'burning out' each year.

In the majority of underperforming athletes, no cause is found and they are diagnosed as suffering from UUPS also known as overtraining syndrome (OTS), chronic fatigue in athletes, sports fatigue syndrome, burnout, staleness or under-recovery syndrome (Figure 11.1; Box 11.1).

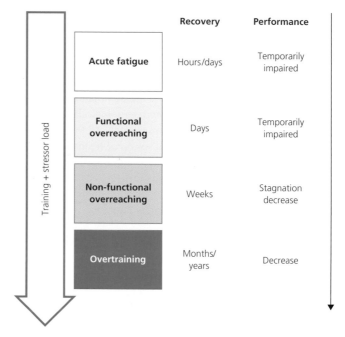

Figure 11.1 The different stages of the overtraining syndrome in the underperforming athlete. Source: Adapted from Meeusen *et al.* 2013. Reproduced by permission of Wolters Kluwer Health

---

Box 11.1 **Precipitating factors of the overtraining syndrome**

- High training load, especially monotonous training or sudden increases in duration or intensity
- High number of competitions
- Other stresses such travelling, unusual environments (heat, altitude) illnesses or injuries and psychological stress of life events, for example exams, moving house or relationship problems.

Symptoms

Underperforming athletes typically present with sports specific decrease in performance, persistent fatigue and mood disturbances. The first duty of the doctor when assessing an athlete with unexplained underperformance is to exclude underlying illness

ABC of Sports and Exercise Medicine, Fourth Edition.
Edited by Gregory P. Whyte, Mike Loosemore and Clyde Williams.
© 2015 John Wiley & Sons, Ltd. Published 2015 by John Wiley & Sons, Ltd.

Box 11.2 **Symptoms of the overtraining syndrome**

- Underperformance
- Depression with loss of motivation, competitive drive and libido
- Increased anxiety and irritability
- Sleep disturbance
- Loss of appetite and weight
- Fatigue
- Frequent minor infections particularly of the upper respiratory tract
- Raised resting pulse rate, decreased heart rate at exhaustion
- Increased symptoms of postural hypotension

Box 11.3 **Exclusion of other causes of chronic fatigue**

- History – enquire about infection, wheeze, eating disorders, chest pain and shortness of breath on exercise
- Examination to exclude a medical cause
- Investigations – these depend on clinical possibilities that may include laboratory tests, lung function and cardiac tests

Box 11.4 **Overtraining may cause immune suppression by:**

- Raised serum cortisol concentrations
- Lower serum glutamine concentrations
- Low-salivary IgA concentrations and saliva volume
- Reduced T-helper/T-suppressor cell ratios

with an appropriate history and examination. Direct questioning often reveals sleep disturbance with difficulty getting to sleep, nightmares, waking in the night or prolonged sleep but waking unrefreshed. Other symptoms are loss of motivation, energy, competitive drive and libido; emotional lability; increased anxiety and irritability; loss of appetite with weight loss or other eating disorders; increased light headiness (postural hypotension) and a raised resting pulse rate, often paired with decreased heart rate at exhaustion. Some athletes suffer from frequent minor infections of the upper respiratory tract (URTI) (Box 11.2).

Distinguishing symptoms

Distinguishing overtraining from normal training fatigue (over reaching) is difficult as the two entities are to be seen as a continuum. Furthermore, both the ability to respond to training and the ability to recover are highly individual features and need to be evaluated on a case-by-case basis, therefore making a universal recommendation of recovery timeframes impossible. Many athletes will be fatigued, irritable, anxious and depressed with increased resting pulse rate and minor infections, but nevertheless recover quickly once the training load has been reduced. Athletes have to train hard in order to improve and the challenge for doctors and sports scientists is to develop reliable measures of recovery so athletes can train as hard as possible but not so hard that they breakdown for many weeks with OTS.

Training

There is often a history of an increase in training load. A common risk factor for the overtraining syndrome is also monotony in training: in some sports such as many endurance disciplines, training is heavy and monotonous and lacks much periodisation (cyclical variation of training). This means that it is more difficult to recover from exercise. The stress of competition and selection pressures may also contribute. Over-trained athletes can usually keep a certain pace for an extended amount of time but describe an inability to lift the pace or sprint for the line.

One swimmer broke the British record and then decided to cut his rest day to train for 7 days a week instead of 6. He broke down after several months and took many weeks to recover. Another swimmer increased his training to 8 h a day. For 4 months his performance improved, but then he started to fail to recover from training. He took months to recover fully.

Nevertheless, it is very rare for athletes to break down after less than 2 weeks of hard training (as in a typical training camp), provided that they then rest and allow themselves to recover afterwards (Box 11.3). This is what happens with normal tapering (=functional overreaching).

Other stressors

In the majority of athletes suffering from unexplained underperformance syndrome, training volume is no different to other athletes, or that of previous years. Adequate recovery is likely to be the critical factor. Stressors such as environmental factors (heat, altitude), excessive travel to training camps or competitions, exams and other life events, poor diet and dehydration will reduce the ability to recover or respond to heavy training.

One rower moved 600 miles to train with a new coach giving up her career and leaving friends and family behind. After 3 months, she developed UUPS despite being used to the level of training and commitment needed. She recovered over 2 months with an appropriate regeneration programme.

Signs

These are inconsistent and generally unhelpful in making the diagnosis because they vary greatly between individuals. The commonly reported signs are increased postural drop in blood pressure and postural rise in heart rate. There is a reduction in sports-specific performance, but laboratory exercise tests might remain unaffected if the right tests are not used. There may also be changes in heart rate variability, increased resting heart rate, impaired post-exercise heart rate recovery, decreased heart rate at exhaustion and increased vulnerability to minor infections (Boxes 11.2 and 11.4).

Investigation

The history and examination should guide t[...] whether further investigations might be he[...] to persuade athletes and coaches of a dia[...] normally some basic screening is neede[...]

that there is no undiagnosed illness. Some serious diseases have presented as UUPS, such as viral myocarditis or cardiac abnormalities, but this is very rare. Prolonged glycogen depletion due to disordered eating (or even eating disorders such as anorexia or bulimia) is a more common cause of fatigue and underperformance. Allergic rhinitis and atopy may present as recurrent URTIs.

Laboratory tests

Laboratory tests are occasionally helpful but cannot be used to make a diagnosis of UUPS (Box 11.5).

Full blood count

Haemoglobin concentrations and packed cell volume decrease as a normal response to heavy training, and athletes reported anaemia is often physiological due to haemodilution and does not affect performance. Such 'pseudo-anaemia' usually resolves after a few days of rest without training.

Iron stores

It is now accepted that low serum ferritin concentrations that reflect iron stores can cause fatigue in the absence of anaemia. Serum ferritin levels may be affected by concurrent illness. The majority of menstruating endurance athletes have ferritins of less than 30 ng/mL which may contribute to fatigue, and this is particularly important if they are considering altitude training. Many Sports and Exercise Medicine doctors recommend taking oral iron (often a liquid preparation since this seems to be better tolerated), and vitamin C to help absorption, to most female endurance athletes who are menstruating.

Viruses

Viral titres are known to show a physiological variance even in healthy athletes, thus, a quantitative assessment is of little use. However, changes in immune status (IgM, IgG, etc.) in comparison to previous investigations for common viruses such as Epstein bar or Cytomegalic virus might be helpful. Nevertheless, identifying a specific virus does not change the management, so is of limited value.

Trace elements and vitamins

It has not been possible to show any link between vitamins, trace elements and UUPS. The widespread use of supplements by athletes does not seem to offer any protection from fatigue and underperformance and should be discouraged due to the risks of contamination with banned substances. Dietary advice should be sought by all athletes, and they must be given strong assurance that a varied diet with sufficient energy negates the

need for supplements in most cases. In the same context, a blood screen for vitamin and mineral status is of little value.

Hormonal assessment

The overtraining syndrome has long been suspected to be a disturbance of the endocrine system. However, to date, there is no validated hormone test to diagnose the condition.

Prevention and early detection

Although by definition UUPS is unexplained, hard training with inadequate recovery is a typical preceding picture. As mentioned, athletes can tolerate different amounts of training and competition stress, so it is difficult for them to differentiate early UUPS from over reaching. Investigators have tried to identify strategies for early detection.

In America, there is about a 10% incidence of 'burnout' among college swimmers that was reduced to zero by daily mood monitoring using a profile of mood state (POMS) questionnaire, by reducing training whenever mood deteriorated and by increasing it when mood improved.

Heart rate

A persistent rise in early morning heart rate, despite rest, is non-specific but does provide objective evidence that something is wrong. The same applies to impaired heart rate recovery after exercise. Heart rate variability has been used for decades by the East European countries to monitor the training status of athletes. Changes in the balance of the activity of the sympathetic and parasympathetic nervous systems occur with hard training and then recovery (with high parasympathetic drive after successful tapering). This may be reflected in heart rate variability giving an objective guide to the extent to recovery. Unfortunately, the changes in athletes with UUPS are very variable, and so heart rate variability cannot be used to make a reliable diagnosis. The heart rate variability seems to change unpredictably as athletes go through fatigue, exhaustion, de-training and recovery. Nevertheless, it is possible that by following individuals over time, a reliable pattern might be obtained.

Other factors

Performance should be monitored carefully and underperformance after a taper is probably most significant. Serial measurements of blood concentrations of haemoglobin and creatine kinase are unlikely to help. It has been shown that a performance decrement of 10% or more in two sequential maximal exercise tests separated by 4 h might indicate OTS.

Prevention requires good diet, full hydration and rest between training sessions. Coaches and athletes must realise that sportspeople with full-time jobs and other commitments will not recover as quickly as those who can relax after training. Periodisation of training should ensure recovery. There is still no reliable objective test to predict which athletes are going to break down after a period of hard training (Box 11.6).

Box 11.6 **Early detection of the overtraining syndrome is difficult. Individual monitoring may help**

- Performance (Rate of perceived exertion, RPE)
- Mood state
- Resting heart rate
- Heart rate recovery after exercise
- Specific exercise testing (test series)

Box 11.7 **Management of the overtraining syndrome**

- Convince coach and athlete of the diagnosis
- Strong reassurance that the prognosis is good
- Relaxation strategies and rest
- Very light exercise, non-discipline specific
- Very short sprints with long rests as condition improves

Management

Sports medicine doctors must work with the coach and the athlete to agree on a recovery programme. The most important task is to persuade both coach and athlete of the diagnosis and that prolonged recovery is needed. Athletes will benefit from a multidisciplinary approach and should see a Sports Dietician and Sports Psychologist if available. Physiologists can also help by setting training levels, a temporary change away from the athlete's specific discipline might often help. During this time, rest and regeneration strategies are essential to recovery and should take the lead on any other training goals (Box 11.7).

Therapeutic exercise

Athletes with UUPS usually show improvement in both performance and mood state with 5 weeks of relative rest. Athletes are advised to exercise aerobically at a level well below training for a few minutes each day and slowly build this up over many weeks. Assuming a central component in the genesis of the overtraining syndrome, it is also advised to cross-train (non-discipline specific) in the beginning, if possible (e.g. an overtrained runner might go for some bicycle rides). The starting level and the increase in training volume will depend on the clinical picture and rate of improvement of the athlete. Recovery can take from weeks to years. Unless held strictly to a recovery programme, many make the mistake of trying to do a normal training session when feeling a little better, suffering from severe fatigue for several days before partially recovering and doing it again.

If an athlete is depressed, anti-depressants and psychological intervention may also be helpful.

Athletes are often surprised at the performance they can produce after 12 weeks of extremely light exercise. It is then that care must be taken not to increase the training load too quickly. When returning to normal training, it is helpful to consider alternating hard and light days of exercise. As they return to full training, athletes are advised to train hard but make sure that they rest and recover completely at least once a week to benefit from all their hard work.

Further reading

Meeusen, R., Duclos, M., Foster, C. *et al.* (2013) Prevention, diagnosis and the treatment of the overtraining syndrome: joint consensus statement of the European College of Sports Science and the American College of Sports Medicine. *Medicine and Science in Sports and Exercise*, **45** (**1**), 186–205.

CHAPTER 12

The Female Athlete Triad

Noel Pollock

Sport & Exercise Medicine, Team Doctor British Athletics, London, UK

OVERVIEW

In this chapter, we describe the female athlete triad. After studying this chapter, the reader will know

- The pathophysiology of the female athlete triad
- The causes of amenorrhea
- The health consequences of the female athlete triad
- Screening and diagnosis of the female athletes triad
- Prevention and treatment of the female athlete triad

Introduction

The 'Female Athlete Triad' is a recognised clinical entity due to the inter-related spectra of energy availability, menstrual function and bone health. It was first described in 1992 as the association between disordered eating, amenorrhoea and osteoporosis and was recognised in athletes participating in sports that emphasised leanness. However, it is now recognised that athletes are distributed along a spectrum with respect to energy availability, menstrual function and bone health and may not manifest the pathological ends of the spectrum at the same time. Therefore, the definition of the female athlete triad has been revised to recognise that athletes may be anywhere along the spectrum of optimal to pathological bone health, menstrual function or energy balance. Clinicians should be aware that detection of dysfunction in one element of the triad should warrant consideration and management of the inter-related spectra. The prevention and management of the female athlete triad is of great importance for those working with female athletes as there is huge potential for negative impact on current and future health and athletic performance.

Pathophysiology of the female athlete triad

The underpinning pathology in the female athlete triad is low-energy availability. This is an essential therapeutic concept as it has

been elegantly shown that it is not the intensity or stress of training that results in the associated menstrual or bone dysfunction, but rather the reduction in energy availability that may be present.

Low-energy availability

Energy availability is defined as the energy remaining for physiological functions after the energy expended during exercise is subtracted from the dietary energy intake. It is important to recognise that this may be advertent or inadvertent. Intense exercise can be an appetite suppressant, and the negative energy balance may be due to inadvertent inadequate refuelling after exercise. In some athletes, energy availability is reduced due to increasing energy expenditure while in others dietary intake may be reduced due to disordered eating. Some athletes may have clinical psychopathological eating disorders, such as anorexia nervosa or bulimia, but while this is important to detect to enable appropriate support it is not usually the case.

Menstrual function

Athletes with aspects of the female athlete triad may present anywhere along the spectrum of eumenorrhoea through oligomenorrhoea (menstrual cycles > 35 days) or amenorrhoea (absence of periods for longer than 3 months). There are numerous causes of amenorrhoea, not related to the female athlete triad, and the clinician should be mindful of other pathological processes that may result in primary or secondary amenorrhoea (Table 12.1).

Loss of periods due to the low-energy availability of the female athlete triad is a functional hypothalamic amenorrhoea. Lutenising

Table 12.1 Causes of amenorrhoea

Anatomical
Uterine pathology or outflow tract disorder
Disorders of sexual differentiation
Endocrine
Hypothalamic (including functional hypothalamic amenorrhoea)
Prolactinoma
Polycystic ovarian syndrome
Other hyperandrogenic disorders (including virilising ovarian tumours)
Cushing's syndrome
Primary ovarian insufficiency
Thyroid dysfunction
Pregnancy

ABC of Sports and Exercise Medicine, Fourth Edition.
Edited by Gregory P. Whyte, Mike Loosemore and Clyde Williams.

hormone secretion from the pituitary gland is disrupted within 5 days of low-energy availability (often defined as $< 30\,\text{kcal}\,\text{kg}^{-1}$ fat-free mass per day). There is a natural variability in women as to the energy availability required to menstruate regularly, but regular menstruation suggests adequate energy is also available for other physiological functions including muscle adaptation, growth and bone remodelling.

Bone health

Bone health is usually assessed by measurement of bone mineral density (BMD) by dual X-ray absorptiometry (DXA). This is only one manifestation of bone health, and cortical thickness and bone geometry are also relevant measures; however, most of the work regarding the female athlete triad has used BMD as the marker of bone health.

Runners, gymnasts and dancers should have increased BMD relative to their peers due to the weight-bearing nature of their regular activity. Indeed often the weight-bearing sites (such as the hip) may be relatively protected with significant deterioration, only noted in less-loaded sites (such as the lumbar spine) or relatively unloaded sites (such as the radius). Therefore, a DXA scan in a female athlete should include four site measurements: whole body, hip, lumbar spine and radius.

Athletes with the female athlete triad may present with normal BMD, low BMD (defined as a Z score between -1 and -2 with secondary risk factors for stress fracture) or osteoporosis (Z-score less than -2 with secondary risk factors for stress fracture). The American College of Sports Medicine and International Society for Clinical Densitometry (ISCD) do not recommend the use of the WHO criteria for the diagnosis of osteoporosis in premenopausal women. The secondary risk factors for fracture include nutritional deficiency, previous history of stress fracture and hypo-oestrogenism.

The primary cause of osteoporosis in postmenopausal women is oestrogen deficiency. This is a high-turnover bone state where oestrogen deficiency results in increased bone resorption. In the female athlete triad, low oestrogen accounts for only a small proportion of abnormal bone remodelling. The female athlete triad is a low-turnover bone state with reduced formation. It is the low-energy availability impact on insulin-like growth factor-1 (IGF-1), growth hormone, cortisol and thyroxine that has more significant impact on bone health than the reduction in oestrogen. For this reason, treatment of the female athlete triad with oestrogen replacement is usually ineffective.

Although bone formation is reduced within several days of low-energy availability, the reductions in BMD may take many months to be recognised on DXA. BMD declines with increasing number of missed menstrual cycles.

Health consequences

Bone health

Athletes with the female athlete triad may have a reduction in BMD that may not be fully reversible. Early intervention is important in adolescent female athletes as 90% of peak bone mass is attained by age 18. As patients reach their peak bone mass around age 30–35, by that time an athlete with the female athlete triad finishes their athletic career; it may be too late to accrue further bone mass. When these athletes reach menopause, their BMD is likely to be severely decreased and the prospect of further bone loss carries a high risk of morbidity.

Stress fractures occur more commonly in athletes with menstrual irregularities, and there is a greater relative risk for stress fracture of two to four times for an amenorrhoeic athlete to a eumenorrhoeic athlete.

Menstrual health

Amenorrhoeic women are usually infertile although, while recovering, they may ovulate before menses return. The consequence of persistent functional hypothalamic amenorrhoea on long-term fertility is not known. Low oestrogen may also result in vaginal dryness, elevated low-density lipoprotein cholesterol and endothelial dysfunction with potential implications for cardiac health.

Eating disorders

Although psychopathological eating disorders are not present in most athletes with the female athlete triad, there are significant health consequences across all body systems if an eating disorder is diagnosed. Anorexia nervosa has a sixfold increase in standard mortality rate and impacts on cardiovascular, renal, endocrine, gastrointestinal and skeletal health.

Screening and diagnosis

Clinicians working with female athletes should be aware of the inter-related spectra and pathophysiology of the female athlete triad. Opportunities should be taken to screen athletes participating in at-risk sports, and when an athlete presents with one aspect of the triad other elements should be investigated. The 2014 Female Athlete Triad Coalition Consensus propose the screening questions listed in Table 12.2. Screening can include nutritional evaluation, menstrual health questionnaires, DXA scanning and blood investigations (Tables 12.3 and 12.4). Causes for amenorrhoea should be thoroughly investigated.

Table 12.2 Annual screening questionnaire

Have you ever had a menstrual period?
How old were you when you had your first menstrual period?
When was your most recent menstrual period?
How many periods have you had in the past 12 months?
Are you presently taking any female hormones?
Do you worry about your weight?
Are you trying to or has anyone recommended that you gain or lose weight?
Are you on a special diet or do you avoid certain types of foods or food groups?
Have you ever had an eating disorder?
Have you ever had a stress fracture?
Have you ever had low-bone density?

Table 12.3 DXA scanning is recommended in the following situations

1. 'High-risk' triad risk factor
Eating disorder
BMI < 17.5 or weight loss > 10% in 1 month
Menarche > 16 years
< 6 menses over 12 months
Two prior stress reactions/fractures or one high-risk stress fracture
Prior Z-score of < 2.0
OR
2. 'Moderate-risk' triad risk factors
Current history of disordered eating for > 6 months
BMI between 17.5 and 18.5
Menarche age 15–16 years
6–8 menses in last 12 months
One prior stress fracture
Prior Z-score between −1.0 and −2.0 (at least 1 year previous to current assessment)
A repeat DXA scan at 1 year is useful to determine the trend of bone mineral density which should be increasing in normal athletes due to increased weight bearing and increasing age

Table 12.4 Appropriate investigations for athlete with features of the female athlete triad

Full blood count
Urea and electrolytes
FSH/LH/oestradiol
Prolactin
Ferritin
Vitamin D
PTH
Thyroid function tests
Serum cortisol
Testosterone and SHBG
US ovaries
DXA scanning

Prevention and treatment

Education of female athletes and their coaches is critical for the prevention of the pathological features of the female athlete triad. Coaches should be cautious about suggesting weight-loss messages to athletes and be aware of the importance of regular menstruation for bone and general health. Athletes are often unaware or sometime unconcerned about long-term health messages. It is important to provide them with this information regularly and also to reinforce the impact of low-energy availability on current athletic performance. While athletes in sports that emphasise leanness, such as endurance running, ballet or gymnastics, may see short-term performance improvement with weight loss, any sustained weight loss and energy deficit is likely to impair performance. It will impact negatively on the ability to adapt and improve from training and increases injury risk to such an extent that the athlete will inevitably spend significant time on the side lines away from their sport. Numerous promising athletic careers have been cut short by recurrent injuries as a result of this condition, and it may be useful for a more senior sportswoman to discuss and educate young athletes on their experience.

The management of athletes with the female athlete triad requires a multidisciplinary approach. A physician who works regularly in sport and with female athletes is ideally placed to coordinate the input of medical, nutritional, psychological and coaching specialists. This may require involvement of a gynaecologist if menstrual dysfunction persists or psychiatrist if features of an eating disorder are present. A clinical nutritionist who can determine and advise on the required energy intake is a critical member of the team.

The first aim of therapy is to increase energy intake or reduce energy expenditure, or a combination of both, to restore a normal menstrual cycle and increase BMD. Energy intake should be a minimum of 2000 kcal per day but often a greater energy intake will be required, depending on expenditure. Increases in body weight are usually required to increase BMD. Adequate amounts of calcium and vitamin D should be in the diet and often additional supplementation is required. There is some research suggesting stress fracture reduction risk in athletes taking regular calcium and vitamin D supplementation. Micronutrient intake including vitamin K, magnesium and zinc is also important. Regular (e.g. weekly) measurement of body weight, in a controlled and standardised manner, is recommended.

Pharmacological therapy, including oestrogen replacement, has not been consistently shown to be efficacious at increasing BMD in this population. It should be emphasised that oestrogen replacement will not normalise the metabolic and hormonal factors that impair bone formation. In addition, commencing these athletes on the OCP means that the athlete and clinician do not get the valuable information of when normal menses is restored. The OCP could be considered with a fracture history and BMD < 2.0 and continues to decrease over 1 year despite non-pharmacological intervention. Transdermal oestradiol (100 µg twice weekly), with cyclical progesterone, may be useful in young athletes without a fracture history, but with BMD < 2.0 to prevent further bone loss although further work is needed.

Bisphosphonates are not recommended in the management of low BMD due to functional hypothalamic amenorrhoea. Their function in limiting bone resorption may slow bone remodelling further and their use in young women may have teratogenic potential due to their long half-life.

Summary

The female athlete triad is recognised as the inter-related spectra of energy availability, menstrual function and bone health. Low-energy availability is the key pathophysiological feature, and correcting energy balance is critical in the management of athletes with these conditions. Prevention, through education and early detection by screening, can have significant impact on athlete's current and long-term health and sustaining athletic performance.

Further reading

American College of Sports Medicine, 401 West Michigan Street, Indianapolis, IN, USA 46202-3233 (www.ACSM.org).

De Souza, M.J., Nattiv, A., Joy, E. et al. (2014) 2014 female athlete triad coalition consensus statement on treatment and return to play of the female athlete triad: 1st international conference held in San Francisco, California, May 2012 and 2nd international conference held in Indianapolis, Indiana, May 2013. *British Journal of Sports Medicine*, **48** (4), 289.

Faculty of Sport & Exercise Medicine (UK). www.fsem.org.uk.

Ihle, R. & Loucks, A.B. (2004) Dose-response relationships between energy availability and bone turnover in young exercising women. *Journal of Bone and Mineral Research: The Official Journal of the American Society for Bone and Mineral Research*, **19** (8), 1231–1240.

Lappe, J., Cullen, D., Haynatzki, G., Recker, R., Ahlf, R. & Thompson, K. (2008) Calcium and vitamin d supplementation decreases incidence of stress fractures in female navy recruits. *Journal of Bone and Mineral Research: The Official Journal of the American Society for Bone and Mineral Research*, **23** (5), 741–749.

Loucks, A.B., Verdun, M. & Heath, E.M. (1998) Low energy availability, not stress of exercise, alters LH pulsatility in exercising women. *Journal of Applied Physiology, Bethesda, Md: 1985*, **84** (1), 37–46.

National Osteoporosis Society, PO Box 10, Radstock, Bath BA3 3YB England (www.nos.org.uk).

CHAPTER 13

The Athlete's Heart

Aneil Malhotra[1], Greg P. Whyte[2] and Sanjay Sharma[3]

[1]Department of Cardiology, St. George's Hospital Medical School, London, UK
[2]Applied Sport & Exercise Science, Research institute for Sport and Exercise Science, Liverpool John Moores University, Liverpool, UK
[3]Cardiologist, Department of Cardiology, St. George's Hospital Medical School, London, UK

OVERVIEW

In this chapter we describe the athlete's heart (AH). After studying this chapter, the reader will know

- Electrocardiographic changes observed in athletes
- Determinants of cardiovascular adaptations to exercise
- The causes of sudden cardiac death in athletes
- Pre-participation screening in athletic populations
- Emergency care for athletes

Introduction

It is well established that participation in at least 4 h of systematic physical activity per week is associated with unique electrical, structural and functional cardiac adaptations that collectively constitute the 'athlete's heart'. These physiological changes are fundamental to the generation and maintenance of a large increase in cardiac output required to meet the demands of repeated bouts of exercise. Although the vast majority of athletes exhibit relatively modest electrical and structural changes, a small proportion may reveal more profound variations that overlap with those observed in individuals who have morphologically mild expressions of several inherited cardiac conditions. Differentiating between physiological cardiac adaption and inherited cardiomyopathies is crucial since an erroneous diagnosis has the potential for serious consequences.

The athlete's ECG

Sinus bradycardia, sinus arrhythmia and early repolarisation changes such as tall T-waves, J-point elevation and concave ST segment elevation are common ECG manifestations of the athlete's heart (AH) (Figure 13.1). First-degree heart block and Mobitz type-I (Wenkbach), second-degree atrioventricular block are also recognised findings in up to 5% of athletes at rest; the majority will revert to sinus rhythm with mild exertion to help the differentiation

between physiological conditioning and cardiac conduction tissue disease. Voltage criteria for left ventricular hypertrophy (LVH) are common, particularly in young males, and do not require further investigation into the absence of symptoms, a positive family history of premature cardiac disease, or accompanying abnormal ECG patterns such as ST-segment depression, pathological Q-waves and left bundle branch block (LBBB); the latter are highly suggestive of a pathological LVH.

In 2010, the European Society of Cardiology (ESC) produced recommendations for the interpretation of a young athlete's ECG. ECG patterns were divided into two categories of common, training-related changes (group 1) and uncommon, training-unrelated changes (group 2). Group 1 patterns do not warrant investigation in the absence of symptoms or a relevant family history. However, in contrast, Group 2 changes should trigger additional diagnostic evaluation to exclude underlying heart disease. More recent criteria have also been published to interpret the athlete's ECG. The ESC and refined criteria are summarised in Figure 13.2.

Repolarisation changes in black athletes (of African/Afro-Caribbean origin)

It is prudent to note that the ESC 2010 ECG recommendations were derived from the Caucasian population and did not take account of the marked repolarisation changes observed in athletes of African or Afro-Caribbean origin (black athletes).

Although T-wave inversion in leads other than III, aVR or V1 are considered abnormal in an adult Caucasian athlete, such ECG patterns are common in black athletes. Indeed, almost 25% of black athletes reveal T-wave inversion. The most common pattern is T-wave inversion confined to leads V1–V4, which is now considered a normal variant. The prevalence of T-wave inversion in the inferior leads and lateral leads is 6% and 4%, respectively. Our own experiences suggest that T-wave inversion in the lateral leads have a positive predictive accuracy of 8% for an underlying cardiomyopathy and always requires comprehensive assessment with echocardiography, cardiac MRI and an exercise stress test.

Echocardiographic changes

On average, young athletes demonstrate a 10–20% increase in left ventricular wall thickness and a 10% increase in left and right

---

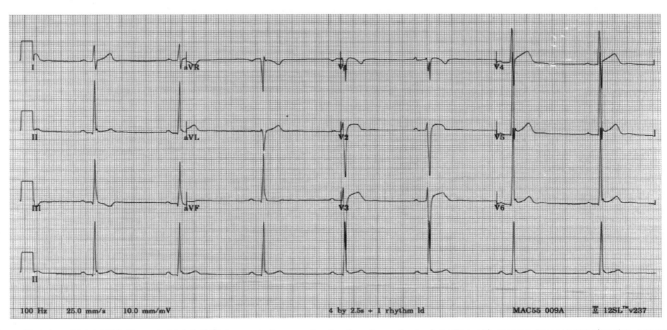

Figure 13.1 An athlete's ECG. Normal athlete's ECG demonstrating a resting bradycardia, early repolarisation with concave ST segment elevation across the precordial leads and isolated QRS voltage criteria for LVH

Common and training-related ECG changes (ESC and Refined Criteria)

- Sinus bradycardia
- First degree atrioventricular block
- Incomplete right bundle branch block
- Early repolarization
- Isolated QRS voltage criteria for LVH

Uncommon and training-unrelated ECG changes (ESC)

- T-wave inversion
- ST-segment depression
- Pathological Q waves
- Left atrial enlargement
- Left axis deviation/ left anterior hemiblock
- Right axis deviation/ left posterior hemiblock
- Ventricular pre-excitation
- Complete left or right bundle branch block
- Long or short corrected QT-interval
- Brugada-like early repolarization

Refined Criteria borderline variants (normal if present in isolation but warranting further investigation if ≥2 present)

- Left/ right atrial enlargement
- Left/ right axis deviation
- Right ventricular hypertrophy
- T-Wave inversion up to V4 in black athletes*

Refined criteria training unrelated changes warranting further investigation

- ST depression
- Pathological Q-waves
- Ventricular pre-excitation
- T wave inversion beyond V1 in white athletes or beyond V4 in black athletes
- Complete left/ right bundle branch block
- QTc ≥470ms in males and ≥480ms in females
- Brugada-like early repolarization
- Atrial or ventricular arrhythmias
- ≥ PVCs per 10 second ECG tracing

Long corrected QT interval >440ms (male, >460ms (female). Short corrected QT interval <380ms. LVH: left ventricular hypertrophy, PVC: premature ventricular complexes. * when preceded by convex ST elevation

Figure 13.2 Classification of common and uncommon findings of the athlete's ECG according to ESC and refined criteria. Long-corrected QT interval > 440 ms (male, > 460 ms (female). Short-corrected QT interval < 380 ms. LVH: left ventricular hypertrophy, PVC: premature ventricular complexes. *When preceded by convex ST elevation

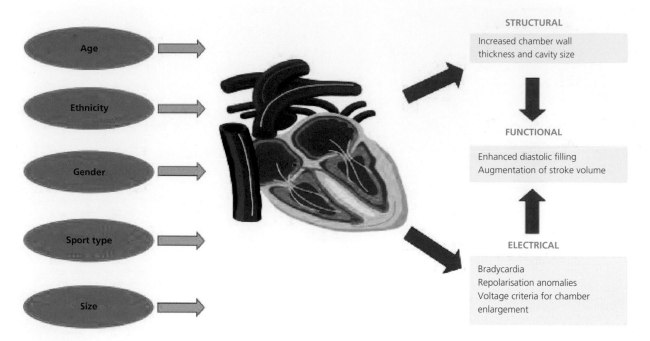

Figure 13.3 Diagram highlighting the influencing factors on cardiac adaptation to exercise

ventricular-end diastolic cavities compared with sedentary controls of similar age and size. Around 50% of athletes reveal left and right ventricular cavity sizes that exceed the upper limit of normal for the general population. In the absence of symptoms or impairment of cardiac function, such athletes do not require further assessment. A left ventricular wall thickness exceeding upper limits for the general population (12 mm) is rare in Caucasian athletes but may be present in 13–18% of male black athletes (up to 15 mm). The differentiation between physiological LVH and morphologically mild hypertrophic cardiomyopathy (HCM) can be particularly challenging in these circumstances.

Determinants of cardiovascular adaptation to exercise

Electrical changes are present in up to 80% of athletes whereas structural changes are observed in 50%. The magnitude with which the electrical and structural changes manifest themselves is determined by a variety of demographic factors and the sporting discipline (Figure 13.3). In general, large adult male athletes develop the greatest increases in cardiac cavity size. Athletes of Afro-Caribbean ethnicity reveal the most profound electrical repolarisation changes (see earlier) and greatest magnitude of left ventricular wall thickness.

The type of sport discipline is an important influencing factor on cardiac adaptation. Pure endurance training, such as long-distance running, is associated with a large preload on the heart and causes a greater cavity dilatation, whereas pure strength training, such as weight-lifting, is associated with a large afterload and has the greatest impact on left ventricular wall thickness. In general, most sports training programmes comprise of both forms of exercise:

therefore, most athletes reveal both an increase in cavity size and wall thickness compared to the sedentary population.

Sudden cardiac death in sport

Cardiac pathology accounts for over 80% of non-traumatic deaths in sport. The incidence of sudden cardiac death (SCD) in sport is approximately 1:50,000. Ninety percentage of deaths occur during or immediately after exercise. Eighty percentage of athletes are asymptomatic prior to death, most of which occur in male athletes and black athletes. Forty percentage of young athletes are aged < 18 at the time of death. The risk of life-threatening ventricular arrhythmias from physical activity in young athletes is nearly three times higher than in non-athletes matched for age. The vast majority of cardiac deaths in young athletes are from hereditary or congenital abnormalities of the heart. The most common cause of death in the United States is HCM, whereas data from Italy report arrhythmogenic right ventricular cardiomyopathy (ARVC) as the commonest cause of death. More recent studies have revealed that the heart may be structurally normal in up to 25% of cases suggesting an ion channel disorder or a congenital accessory pathway as a potential cause. The causes of SCD in young athletes are shown in Figure 13.4

The grey zone: AH or cardiomyopathy

A common conundrum faced by the sports physician is the differentiation between physiological LVH and morphologically mild HCM, in instances where the left ventricular wall thickness is between 12 and 16 mm. In most situations, the differentiation is possible based on symptoms, a family history, the 12-lead ECG and echocardiogram. A small number of athletes may require

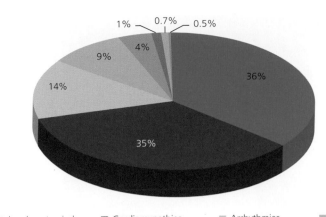

Figure 13.4 Causes of sudden cardiac death in young athletes (%). Data from Papadakis *et al.*, "Preparticipation screening for cardiovascular abnormalities in young competitive athletes"

■ Congenital and anatomical ■ Cardiomypathies ■ Arrhythmias ■ Infectious
■ Degenerative ■ Undetermined ■ Acquired ■ "Normal heart"

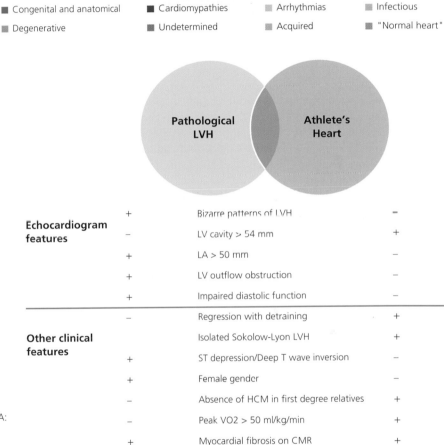

	Pathological LVH		Athlete's Heart
Echocardiogram features	+	Bizarre patterns of LVH	−
	−	LV cavity > 54 mm	+
	+	LA > 50 mm	−
	+	LV outflow obstruction	−
	+	Impaired diastolic function	−
Other clinical features	−	Regression with detraining	+
		Isolated Sokolow-Lyon LVH	+
	+	ST depression/Deep T wave inversion	−
	+	Female gender	−
	−	Absence of HCM in first degree relatives	+
	−	Peak VO2 > 50 ml/kg/min	+
	+	Myocardial fibrosis on CMR	+

Figure 13.5 Practical diagnostic algorithm for differentiating athlete's heart from morphologically mild HCM in athletes with a left ventricular wall thickness of 12–16 mm. CMR: cardiac magnetic resonance imaging; LA: left atrium; LV: left ventricle; LVH: left ventricular hypertrophy; VO$_2$ max: maximum oxygen uptake

additional investigations in the form of a cardiopulmonary exercise test and a cardiac MRI.

In a male athlete with an unexplained left ventricular wall thickness of > 12 mm, the presence of cardiac symptoms, a family history of HCM, bizarre patterns of LVH, a small left ventricular cavity, abnormal diastolic function or the presence of pathological Q waves, ST segment depression or LBBB favour HCM over AH (Figure 13.5).

Cardiac MRI may provide additional information with better visualisation of the left ventricular apex and lateral wall. Specialist techniques such as the use of gadolinium may reveal underlying fibrosis within the myocardium, which would be suggestive of HCM. The right ventricle may also be visualised more clearly to help identify pathologies such as ARVC.

In cases of uncertainty, despite comprehensive evaluation a period of detraining may resolve the diagnostic dilemma; the resolution LVH would be consistent with AH. However, most athletes are reluctant to detrain as it costs fitness and team selection. Figure 13.5 illustrates a clinical algorithm to help differentiate between the so-called 'grey zone' of pathological LVH from HCM in athletes and physiological LVH from exercise adaptation.

Pre-participation screening in young athletes

The ESC and many sporting bodies including the Lawn Tennis Association, Football Association, the English Institute of Sport and the International Olympic Committee advocate pre-participation

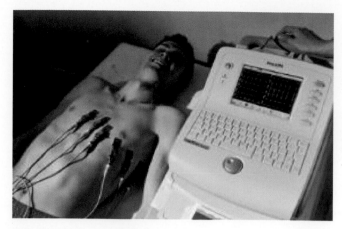

Figure 13.6 A young athlete undergoing a pre-participation ECG (image courtesy of cardiac risk in the young charity)

screening of all young competitive athletes with a health questionnaire, physical examination and 12-lead ECG (Figure 13.6). Such practice is usually confined to the most elite athletes in many developed countries and has been shown to identify athletes with potentially serious cardiac diseases. Indeed data from Italy, where pre-participation screening is mandatory, has shown an incredible reduction in death rates from 3.6/100,000 to 0.4/100,000. However, despite these impressive figures, there are many issues with ECG screening including a high false positive rate based on current ECG interpretation criteria, a false negative rate of around 15% and the lack of resources and infrastructure to develop a *de novo* large-scale screening programme for all athletes in most countries.

Emergency medical care and the athlete

Given that pre-participation screening may fail to identify all athletes at risk of SCD, it is prudent that trained personnel are available at sporting events to promptly recognise cardiac arrest and institute advanced life support measures. Such measures have improved survival rates from cardiac arrest by at least threefold. An efficient and coordinated response to cardiac emergencies includes the following: personnel as first responders trained in cardiopulmonary resuscitation; the provision of external automated external defibrillators; coordinating communication and transportation systems and ensuring access to appropriate medical equipment and supplies.

Further reading

Drezner, J.A., Ackerman, M.J., Anderson, J. *et al.* (2013) Electrocardiographic interpretation in athletes: the 'Seattle criteria'. *British Journal of Sports Medicine*, **47** (**3**), 122–124.

Papadakis, M., Whyte, G. & Sharma, S. (2008) Preparticipation screening for cardiovascular abnormalities in young competitive athletes. *British Medical Journal*, **337**, a1596.

Papadakis, M., Carre, F., Kervio, G. *et al.* (2011) The prevalence, distribution, and clinical outcomes of electrocardiographic repolarization patterns in male athletes of African/Afro-Caribbean origin. *European Heart Journal*, **32** (**18**), 2304–23013.

Sheikh, N. & Sharma, S. (2011) Overview of sudden cardiac death in young athletes. *The Physician and Sportsmedicine*, **39** (**4**), 22–36.

Whyte, G. & George, K. (2012) Exercise and the heart. *Dialogues in Cardiovascular Medicine*, **17** (**1**), 7–30.

Zaidi, A., Ghani, S., Sharma, R. *et al.* (2013) Physiological right ventricular adaptation in elite athletes of African and Afro-Caribbean origin. *Circulation*, **127** (**17**), 1783–92.

CHAPTER 14

Extreme Temperature Sport and Exercise Medicine

Michael J. Tipton

Human and Applied Physiology, Extreme Environments Laboratory, DSES, University of Portsmouth, Portsmouth, UK

OVERVIEW

In this chapter the influence of the thermal environment is reviewed. Despite the fact that this influence can range from subtle impairments of performance to death, it is surprisingly ill-considered and prepared for by many sportspeople. Whilst understanding of the impact of heat on performance and health has risen with high profile poor performances in warm environments, few understand the risks associated with cold, and ways of minimising them. Fewer still understand conditions like non-freezing cold injury. This chapter outlines the responses to hot and cold environments and ways of assessing and minimising the associated risks and their impact on performance.

Introduction

Since the 5th century BC, when Herodicus was advocating good diet for physical training, the influence of nutrition on sporting performance has been a predominant and enduring theme. In contrast, the influence of the environment is a relatively recent consideration, and one that is often overlooked despite the fact that environmental stress can have an enormous impact on performance and safety. Over the last 20 years more than 100 American footballers have died from excessive heat stress. Fifty-six percent (212) of the UK's immersion-related deaths in 2012, which were not crime nor suicide related, resulted from sporting activities; making immersion, by a long way, the leading cause of death of sportspeople undertaking their sport.

In August 2016, the summer Olympics will take place in Rio de Janeiro when peak air temperature averages 27 °C, exceeding 32 °C or dropping below 24 °C 1 day in 10. Relative humidity ranges from 54% to 97% over the course of a typical August. Even these Southern Hemisphere winter climatic conditions are sufficient to cause impairment of some elite sporting activities. In this chapter, the influence of heat, cold and altitude on the body is reviewed.

ABC of Sports and Exercise Medicine, Fourth Edition.
Edited by Gregory P. Whyte, Mike Loosemore and Clyde Williams.
© 2015 John Wiley & Sons, Ltd. Published 2015 by John Wiley & Sons, Ltd.

Temperature

Thermal balance

Heat is exchanged between the body and the environment by four physical processes convection (C), conduction (K), radiation (R) and evaporation (E). In order to remain in thermal balance, the heat being gained by the body must equal that being lost, such that no heat is stored (S) in the body. This can be expressed in the heat balance equation as

$$M - (W) = R \pm C \pm K - E$$

where the unit for each term is $W\,m^{-2}$, M is the metabolic energy utilisation (metabolic rate) and W is the measurable external work.

The catabolic chemical reactions of the body liberate energy; the sum total of which constitutes total metabolic energy utilisation or rate (M). The biggest cause of variation in energy expenditure comes with muscle activity such as exercise or shivering. Only a maximum of 25% of the chemical energy used during muscular contraction is converted into mechanical work, the remainder is liberated as heat; during sustained vigorous exercise, heat production can reach in excess of 20 kcal min^{-1}. If the body were prevented from losing any of the heat it produced, a fatal level of heat storage would be reached in about 4 h when at rest, and after just 25 min with moderate exercise.

The thermoregulatory system of the body is a complex mix of cold and warm receptors, afferent and efferent pathways, central nervous system integrating and controlling centres, and effectors. The primary aim of this system is to maintain body temperature within safe limits. In air at 25–28 °C, or water at 35 °C, a naked, resting individual can maintain body temperature by varying the amount of heat delivered to the skin via the circulation, in this situation cutaneous blood flow averages 250 ml min^{-1}. As air/water temperature falls or increases, shivering or sweating must be initiated in an attempt to defend body temperature. These autonomic responses are costly in terms of substrate or fluid and have only a limited capability to defend body temperature when compared to behaviour (e.g. clothing, housing and heating).

Whenever possible in air, body temperature is kept within about 1 °C of 37 °C and skin temperature averages 33 °C. Humans can survive a fall in core temperature increase of about 10 °C (this figure can vary dramatically) and an increase in about 6 °C.

Heat

Human skin contains 2–4 million sweat glands, more per unit area than any other mammal. The sweat glands are activated within seconds of the commencement of exercise in a warm environment and reach maximum output after about 30 min. Sweat is a hypotonic saline solution (0.3–0.6% NaCl). In a hot environment (above body temperature), heat produced by metabolism and that gained by K, C and R must be matched by that lost by E. This emphasises the importance of the evaporation of sweat in a hot environment.

Evaporation of sweat

No sweat can evaporate when relative humidity (rh) is 100% (air at skin temperature, saturated with water vapour).
  The rate of evaporation depends on the following:

- Skin surface area that is wet.
- Difference between the water vapour pressure at the skin surface (P_s) and that in the air (P_a).
- Air movement around the body (wind or body movement); in still air, the water vapour pressure next to the skin rises as sweat is produced and lowers the gradient between P_s and P_a.

The fact that P_s can still be greater than P_a when ambient temperature is higher than mean skin temperature is the physical basis for evaporation being the only route for heat loss in a hot environment.
  It is not sweat production, but sweat evaporation that cools the body. As a consequence, a temperate humid environment (or microclimate such as under clothing) can represent just as large a threat as a hot dry environment. Heat-related deaths have occurred in American footballers in 23.9 °C and 95% rh. It is important to assess an environment in terms of its air temperature, humidity and radiant heat load. This can be achieved using the wet bulb-globe temperature (WBGT) index.

It is normal for the deep body temperature of an individual to increase to a new steady-state level during exercise in air. This is thought to be a regulated rise that is similar in magnitude between individuals when they work at the same relative work load (%VO_{2max}), and represents an adjustment that optimises metabolic function. The body temperature attained during exercise is dependent on work rate (up to 65% VO_{2max}), but independent of ambient conditions over a range of temperatures (5–25 °C) with relatively low humidity ('Prescriptive Zone'). Above the prescriptive zone deep body temperature rises and may, or may not, plateau at a higher temperature depending on whether or not the overall heat load is 'compensable' by the thermoregulatory system (Figure 14.1).

Heat: effects on performance

Exercise in the heat places an additional strain on the cardiovascular system. Heat dissipation during moderate to severe exercise in the heat occurs more by repartitioning cardiac output than by increasing it; 15–25% of cardiac output is directed to the skin to assist in heat loss, constriction of splanchnic and renal vascular beds enables the majority of this increase in cutaneous blood flow. Heart rate is

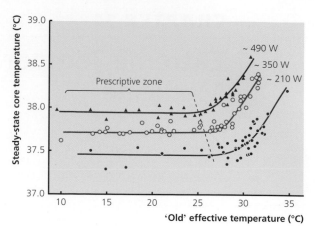

Figure 14.1 The prescriptive zone (Lind, "A physiological criterion for setting thermal environmental limits for everyday work". Source: Lind, 1963. Reproduced with permission from American Physiological Society). Effective temperature is the temperature of still, unsaturated air that gives rise to an equivalent thermal sensation as that evoked in other environments with different temperatures and humidities

unable to offset the fall in stroke volume during maximal exercise in the heat; as a consequence, maximal cardiac output falls. This severely limits the ability of unacclimatised individuals to exercise in such conditions. VO_{2max} is usually reported to be lower in hot than temperate climates.

Submaximal exercise performance can also be affected: marathon performance declines by about 1 min for each 1 °C increase in air temperature above 15°C. Compromised muscle blood flow, plus decreased hepatic blood flow, results in an earlier onset of anaerobic metabolism and blood lactate accumulation. Muscle glycogen utilisation is increased (substrate for anaerobic metabolism), and fatigue occurs earlier during prolonged moderate exercise in the heat. There is also a diminished central drive to exercise in hyperthermic individuals. Heating does not decrease maximum strength but does reduce muscle endurance and time to fatigue.

Given that thermoneutral water temperature for moderate exercise is about 25 °C, open water swimming events in warmer water also present the risk of hyperthermia, particularly with a co-existent radiant heat load and due, in part, to the limited ability to lose heat by the evaporation of sweat. Warm water swimming has resulted in heat illness and claimed a life in recent years.

Aerobically fit individuals are able to perform for longer time in hot environments, and tolerate higher levels of hyperthermia than less fit individuals due, in part, to their larger blood volume and greater sweating capacity. However, abnormally high core temperatures impair exercise performance in all individuals in the heat.

Cardiovascular responses of unacclimatised men walking for 15 min at 10% gradient in 26 and 43 °C

	Response at 43 °C compared to 26 °C
Central blood volume	16% lower
Oxygen consumption	Same
Heart rate	15% higher
a-VO_2 difference	No significant difference
Stroke volume	Same

Dehydration during exercise in the heat

During exercise body fluid loss, primarily due to sweating, increases by an amount that depends on several factors including environmental temperature, fitness, level of acclimatisation, intensity and duration of the activity. An athlete training in a hot climate may require $4\text{--}12\,l\,d^{-1}$. Without adequate fluid replacement, sportsmen can lose body fluid equivalent to 3–10% of their body mass while exercising.

In comparison with the responses seen when hydrated, fluid loss equivalent to 5% of body mass increases rectal temperature due to decreased sweating and cutaneous blood flow. Dehydration between 1.9 and 4.3% of body mass can reduce endurance by 22–48% and VO_{2max} by 10–22%. The risk of heat illness is increased if exercise is undertaken in the heat in a dehydrated state.

Heat illness

The problems caused by heat result from decreased circulating blood volume and consequent alterations in regional blood flow; increased blood viscosity; and a direct effect of temperature on the respiratory centres and proteins. Heat illness can occur in cool or temperate conditions if humidity is high, or individuals are unable to offload the heat produced from high work rates due to clothing.

A large list of factors influence thermoregulation and an individual's susceptibility to heat illness, these include the following:

- Air temperature, humidity, movement, radiant heat load
- Body size (mass, body surface area, skinfold thickness) – heat stroke occurs 3.5 times more frequently in excessively overweight young adults than in individuals of average body mass
- State of training/sudden increase in training (military recruits with low aerobic fitness [> 12 min for 1.5 mile run] and a high body mass index [$> 26\,kg\,m^{-2}$] have a ninefold greater risk of heat illness)
- Degree of acclimatisation
- Hydration status
- Heat production (exercise intensity/duration)
- Clothing worn (vapour permeability, fit, colour)
- State of health (e.g. fever – viral illness, cold, flu; diabetes mellitus, cardiovascular disease, gastroenteritis/diarrhoea)
- Genetic disorders (e.g. mutations for cystic fibrosis, malignant hyperthermia)
- Skin disorders, including sunburn over 5% of body surface area
- Use of medication (e.g. diuretics; antihistamines; ergogenic stimulants)
- Sweat gland dysfunction (e.g. prickly heat)
- Salt depletion
- Age
- Sleep deprivation
- Glycogen or glucose depletion
- Acute/chronic alcohol/drug abuse

Because some of these factors can operate acutely (e.g. infection), an individual may suffer heat illness in circumstances in which they were previously unaffected.

Heat illness

Heat cramps. Usually occur in the specific muscles exercised due to an imbalance in the body's fluid volume and electrolyte concentration, and low energy stores. Core temperature remains in normal range. Aetiology unknown. Can be prevented by an appropriate rehydration strategy and treated by stretching and massage.

Heat exhaustion. The most common form of heat illness, defined as the inability to continue exercise in the heat. Usually seen in unacclimatised individuals. Caused by ineffective circulatory adjustments and reduced blood volume. Characterised by breathlessness, hyperventilation, weak and rapid pulse, low blood pressure, dizziness, headache, flushed skin, nausea, paradoxical chills, irritability, lethargy and general weakness. Deep body temperature is raised, but not excessively, sweating persists and there is no organ damage. Heat exhausted individuals should stop exercising, lie down, control breathing if hyperventilating and rehydrate; failure to do so can result in progression to severe heat illness. Heat exhaustion is a predominant problem when body water loss exceeds 7% of body mass.

Heat stroke. Medical emergency resulting from failure of the thermoregulatory system as a result of a high deep body temperature (> 40.5 °C). Characterised by confusion, absence of sweating, hot and dry skin, circulatory instability. If not treated by immediate cooling, results in death from circulatory collapse and multi-organ damage. Aggressive steps should be taken to cool the casualty as mortality is related to the degree and duration of hyperthermia. Consider using 'artificial sweat' (this involves spraying with tepid water/alcohol solution) and fanning to enhance evaporation; fluid replacement (do not over-infuse/overload; can result in pulmonary oedema). Consider colder water immersion/ice packs for those without a peripheral circulation.

Heat stroke should be the working diagnosis in anyone who has an altered mental state. Deep body temperature should be monitored every 5 min; deep (15 cm) rectal temperature is preferable to mouth or ear canal as these may be influenced by hyperventilation and/or the active cooling strategy employed. Heat-exhausted individuals should improve rapidly with appropriate immediate care. Any individuals who do not improve quickly should be evacuated to the next level of medical care.

Long-term recovery from exertional heat stroke is idiosyncratic and in severe cases may take up to a year.

Exertional rhabdomyolysis. This is caused by muscle damage resulting in the release of cellular contents (e.g. myoglobin, potassium, phosphate, creatine kinase and uric acid) into the circulation. More likely if dehydrated or taking non-steroidal anti-inflammatory drugs. Overt signs include muscle pain, tenderness and weakness, very dark urine. Treat by giving fluids, evacuate to intensive medical care, kidney function should be assessed.

Strategies to maintain performance in the heat and avoid heat illness

Maintaining fluid balance

It is important to recognise the signs of dehydration, which include fatigue, headache, irritability, dark urine and insomnia. Clearly it is disadvantageous to begin exercise in the heat in a dehydrated state. It is not possible to 'adapt' to low water intake and this should not be attempted. However, there does appear to be significant inter-individual differences in the susceptibility to dehydration.

The upper rate at which fluid will empty from the stomach during exercise is 1–1.5 l per hour; even the most effective oral fluid replacement strategies will fail to prevent dehydration above this level of sweat loss. Volitionally, most individuals replace only about half of the fluid they need to rehydrate, as thirst is quenched at this level of rehydration.

The general principles of fluid replacement are as follows:

- Because sweat is hypotonic in comparison with body fluids, water rather than mineral replacement is the primary concern.
- Water absorption occurs mainly in the upper part of the small intestine and depends on osmotic gradients. Adding small amounts of glucose and sodium to a rehydration drink has little negative effect on gastric emptying. The presence of glucose may accelerate fluid uptake due to the active co-transport of glucose and sodium across the intestinal mucosa. Adding sodium will help to maintain plasma sodium concentrations, reduce urine output and sustain the sodium-dependent osmotic drive to drink.
- Drinks with low-sugar content (2–4%, 20–40 g l^{-1}) will not supply much energy, but if they are hypotonic and have high-sodium content (40–60 mmol l^{-1}, 1–1.5 g l^{-1}) they will give the fastest water replacement. The fastest rate of energy supply is achieved with high-sugar concentrations (15–20%, 150–200 g l^{-1}), but this limits the rate at which water is absorbed.
- Gastric emptying slows when ingested fluids have high osmolality (plasma osmolality = 280 mOsm l^{-1}) or caloric content. A drink containing glucose polymers rather than simple sugars minimises this negative effect.
- Gastric volume influences gastric emptying, with emptying rate increasing with volume in the stomach. Consuming 400–600 ml immediately before exercise optimises the transfer of fluids into the intestine. Drinking 150–250 ml at 15 min intervals during exercise maintains gastric volume and fluid uptake at maximal levels of about 1–1.5 l per hour.
- A drink that tastes good and is cool is more likely to be drunk.
- Highly carbonated beverages retard gastric emptying.

Overhydration and hyponatraemia

Athletes should not drink as much as they can in the belief that more is better. Concerns about excessive overhydration and hyponatraemia (low blood sodium) among endurance athletes has led the USA Track & Field (governing body) to urge runners to hydrate based on individual need. One post-race study of 481 participants in the 2002 Boston Marathon suggested that 13% experienced hyponatraemia, one female participant died from hyponatraemic encephalopathy. This is somewhat higher than the 0.31% reported following the 2000 Houston Marathon. Nevertheless, it is a condition that, according to descriptions in the medical literature, has been responsible for at least 7 deaths and 250 cases.

Risk factors include the following: being a female runner with slow finishing times in long duration events (running speed < 5 mph); excessive fluid consumption (15 l in 5–6 h of exercise); and under-replacement of sodium losses.

Hyponatraemia can result in intracellular swelling that, if severe enough, can produce symptoms of central nervous dysfunction, lung congestion and muscle weakness. Hyponatraemia and dehydration-mediated heat exhaustion share many symptoms, and laboratory tests are required to distinguish between the two. Patients with dehydration-mediated heat exhaustion respond fairly quickly to fluid replacement, whereas the condition of those with hyponatraemia will be aggravated by the administration of hypotonic fluids.

The International Marathon Medical Directors Association (IMMDA, 2002) stated that blanket hydration recommendations for athletes are incorrect and unsafe, and that they should drink as needed but not exceed 400–800 ml per hour: lesser amounts for slower, smaller athletes in mild environments, greater amounts for faster athletes in warmer environments.

Bodycooling

The benefit of whole-body pre-cooling appears to be dependent on environment and activity. It has not been found to be beneficial in simulated triathlons or soccer-related activities under normal environments. In contrast, pre-cooling to reduce core temperature by 0.7 °C (e.g. immersion in cool [23 °C] water) has been shown to increase subsequent exercise endurance in hot and humid conditions, with time to exhaustion being inversely related to initial body temperature. Just cooling the skin by 5–6 °C reduces thermal strain and increases cycling performance (distance cycled in 30 min) in warm and humid conditions. A recent approach is the use of ice–slurry ingestion to cool; this method has the benefit of also helping to maintain hydration and has been favourably compared with cold water ingestion in hot (34 °C) conditions.

Returning body temperature to normal levels between repeated bouts of exercise in the heat helps to maintain performance, decreases physiological strain and extends work time. Two of the quickest and simplest ways of doing this for those in lightweight sports attire and with a peripheral circulation (i.e. not suffering heat stroke) is by whole body fanning and/or hand immersion in cold water. The rates of heat exchange achieved by these methods compare favourably with those achieved by the use of ice vests or air-perfused vests.

The use of ice-cold water immersions after training and competition as a recovery aid has become increasingly popular. Those advocating such cryotherapy for recovery from exercise cite subjective responses and its ability to blunt inflammation by reducing local metabolism and inducing vasoconstriction. However, the lack of appropriate controls and measures of muscle temperatures, and the wide variety of exercise protocols undertaken in the scientific literature on this topic have resulted in general disagreement about the utility of cryotherapy in terms of the most appropriate methodology and type of exercise that might benefit from it. Indeed, it remains possible that this intervention is often no more beneficial than conventional post-exercise strategies (e.g. light exercise 'warm down'). The possible hazardous consequences of post-exercise immersions in ice-cold water, such as non-freezing cold injury (NFCI), are usually ignored when this intervention is assessed.

Acclimatisation

Repeated exposure to hot environments that produce increases in deep body and skin temperature and profuse sweating result in acclimatisation to heat; this improves exercise capacity and comfort in the heat, and possibly also in temperate environments. It is important to exercise during these exposures (gradually increasing exercise intensity each day until at normal pace), as resting in the heat provides only partial acclimatisation. The acclimatisation acquired is specific to the climate and activity level; those acclimatised to hot dry environments will require additional time to acclimatise if they move to hot humid environments.

The process requires exposure to representative environmental temperatures for at least 2 h per day and takes a total of 10–14 days. No more than 3 days should elapse between successive exposures. The adjustments to the raised body temperatures associated with exercise mean that fitter individuals can acclimatise more quickly (7–10 days). However, even fit individuals need to exercise in a hot environment in order to achieve full acclimatisation.

The exposures can be in the field (acclimatisation) or in a suitable climatic chamber (acclimation). Using sweat suits (impermeable/semi-permeable clothing) or saunas is partially effective. The beneficial changes associated with heat acclimatisation include the following:

- Sensitivity to, and secretion of, aldosterone increases. This increases sodium and chloride reabsorption in sweat ducts and renal tubules, which results in lowered salt content in sweat (e.g. sweat sodium reduced from 50 to 25 mmol l^{-1}) and increased osmotic retention of water. The increased plasma volume that is produced is responsible for many of the secondary benefits of heat acclimatisation.
- Less cardiovascular strain.
- More effective distribution of cardiac output.
- Improved cutaneous blood flow.
- Earlier onset and greater rate of sweating.
- More effective distribution of sweat over the skin surface.
- Lower skin and deep body temperatures for a given level of exercise.
- Improved physical work capacity.
- Increased comfort.
- Decreased reliance on carbohydrate metabolism.

Because an acclimatised individual can produce more sweat, they have a greater fluid requirement in order to maintain hydration. On return to a temperate climate, the major benefits of heat acclimatisation are retained for a week, 75% are then lost within 3 weeks.

Assessing the risk of a warm air environment

The most widely used of the heat stress indices is the WBGT index, the formula for which is:

$$WBGT = 0.1T_{db} + 0.7T_{wb} + 0.2T_g$$

where T_{db} is the dry bulb temperature, T_{wb} is the wet bulb temperature and T_g is the globe temperature. The weightings emphasise the importance of humidity for heat stress.

WBGT meters can be purchased and are relatively inexpensive. They consist of a thermometer/thermistor (dry bulb): a thermometer/thermistor covered with a dampened wick (wet bulb), and a thermometer/thermistor enclosed on a black metal sphere that absorbs radiant energy from the surroundings (globe temperature).

Recommendations. To reduce the chance of heat injury in athletic activity in lightly clothed individuals:

WBGT	
26.5–28.8	Use discretion, especially if untrained or unacclimatised
29.5–30.5	Avoid strenuous activity
> 31.2	Avoid exercise training

For those sportsmen wearing heavier clothing, the lower temperature in each range should be used.

The American College of Sports Medicine WBGT recommendations for continuous activities such as running and cycling.

< 18 °C	Low risk
18–23 °C	Moderate risk
23–28 °C	High risk. Those with predisposing factors for heat illness (see main text) should not compete
> 28 °C	Very high risk. Postpone competition

The optimum temperature for prolonged strenuous exercise (cycle ergometry), as assessed by time to exhaustion, is 11 °C. Exercise time is reduced by 13% at 21 °C and 45% at 31 °C.

Psychological interventions

A comparatively recent innovation has been the use of psychological skills training (PST) to try and alter performance in the heat and cold. Originally designed to improve performance on discrete skills in highly competitive environments, PST has now been shown to improve running performance in the heat and breath-hold time in cold water. PST is most effective for altering responses that are under conscious control, such as selecting a pace at which to exercise, terminating exercise or the break of breath-holding.

Clothing in the heat

To minimise the thermal burden, clothing should be the following:

- Lightweight: to minimise insulation and increase the exchange of air between the microclimate (beneath the clothing) and environment with body movement ('Bellows effect').
- Light coloured: to reflect more radiant heat.
- Loose: to facilitate the Bellows effect.
- Vapour permeable: to facilitate evaporative heat loss.
- Made from materials (e.g. linen or cotton) that readily absorb water: to facilitate evaporative heat loss.

Wearing protective clothing for sporting activities can impose a significant thermal load on the body and result in significantly higher skin and deep body temperatures. The combination of insulative clothing and high levels of metabolic heat production has resulted in cases of fatal heat stroke.

Cold

Although air temperature can fall to lower levels than water temperature, it is water that represents the greater threat because of its higher thermal conductivity and specific heat. This helps to explain why, in the United Kingdom, cold water immersion is the largest killer of sportspeople undertaking their sport (221 sports-related immersion deaths in 2012).

In most circumstances in air, the heat produced by exercise is sufficient to offset that lost to a cold environment, particularly when combined with the careful use of clothing. In air, therefore, problems with deep body cooling tend to only arise when heat production is reduced due to injury or exhaustion. In contrast, exercise tends to accelerate rather than prevent cooling in cold water because the heat produced by exercise does not balance the increased heat lost resulting from moving in the water and increased blood flow to the exercising peripheral musculature.

Cold: effects on performance

In air or water, the first tissue to be affected on exposure to cold is the skin. Skin cooling is accentuated by the peripheral vasoconstriction initiated by the body in order to reduce heat loss. It is the extremities (hands and feet) that are most affected due to their high surface area-to-mass ratio, and the fact that their major source of heat, blood flow, has been restricted by vasoconstriction. This, in part, explains why it is the extremities that normally receive cold injuries.

Rapid skin cooling on immersion in cold water evokes 'Cold shock', a set of cardiorespiratory responses that include uncontrollable hyperventilation, hypertension and increased cardiac workload, which can be precursors to cardiovascular accidents and drowning. In situations where the face is also immersed, co-activation of sympathetic and parasympathetic inputs to the heart can produce 'Autonomic Conflict' resulting in arrhythmias

that can be the precursor to sudden death in a variety of sporting situations including open water swimming; 79% of those who die during triathlons do so during the swim. Indeed, approximately 60% of those that die on immersion in cold water generally do so within the first minutes of immersion, long before hypothermia can occur.

The cold shock response subsides after 2–3 min and the next tissues to cool are the superficial nerves and muscles. This can result in physical incapacitation in as little as 15 min in water; the time taken for this to occur depends on the exact nature of the environment (air/water, temperature, wind speed). The conduction of action potentials is slowed ($15\,\text{m s}^{-1}$ per $10\,^{\circ}\text{C}$ fall in local temperature) and their amplitude reduced. Below a muscle temperature of $27\,^{\circ}\text{C}$, the contractile force and rate of force application are reduced and fatigue occurs earlier – maximum power output falls by 3% per degree celsius fall in muscle temperature. As a consequence, speed of movement, dexterity, strength and mechanical efficiency are all reduced with cooling.

Despite the fact that the deep body temperature of an individual immersed in cold water will cool about four times faster than when in air at the same temperature, for adult humans hypothermia does not occur within 30 min of head-out immersion in even the coldest water temperatures. When it does occur, a fall in deep body temperature intensifies shivering, which raises oxygen consumption during submaximal exercise (e.g. 9% in water at $25\,^{\circ}\text{C}$; 25.3% in water at $18\,^{\circ}\text{C}$). The increase is greater in leaner individuals. Thus, the energy cost of submaximal exercise is increased in water cooler than $26\,^{\circ}\text{C}$; this can result in a more rapid depletion of carbohydrate and lipid energy sources and earlier onset of fatigue (Figure 14.2).

When shivering occurs during exercise in the cold, cardiac output is elevated above levels seen during exercise in temperate conditions. Stroke volume is usually higher and heart rate lower during exercise in the cold, due to increased central blood volume and cardiac preload as a result of peripheral vasoconstriction (and increased hydrostatic squeeze when in water).

VO_{2max}, during ergometry or swimming, and maximum performance are both reduced during cold water immersion. This

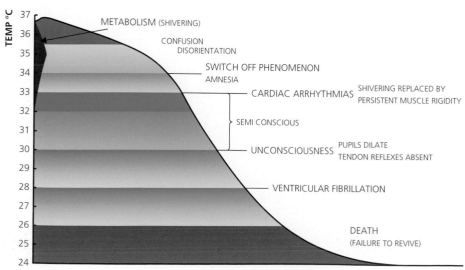

Figure 14.2 Signs and symptoms of hypothermia (from Golden, 1973 in Golden and Tipton, 2002, *Essentials of Sea Survival*. Reproduced with permission of SAGE Publications Ltd) NB. Human Kinetics published The Essentials of Sea Survival

reduction occurs in water with a temperature as high as 25 °C and is approximately linearly related to deep body temperature, with a 10–30% reduction observed following a 0.5–2 °C fall in deep body temperature. Associated with this reduction in VO_{2max}, lactate appears in the blood at lower workloads and accumulates at a more rapid rate than in thermoneutral conditions. This suggests that oxygen delivery to the working muscles may be reduced during profound cooling. This situation may be accentuated by a left shift in the oxygen dissociation curve with cooling. A decrease in deep body temperature of 0.5–1.5 °C results in a reduction of 10–40% in the capacity to supply oxygen to meet the increased requirements of activity. With more profound cooling, anaerobic metabolism is also reduced due to muscle cooling and direct impairment of the processes responsible for the anaerobic production of energy.

Dehydration is common in cold environments because thirst is blunted, water is not always easily available (frozen) and respiratory water loss can be high in cold dry environments. Furthermore, cold exposure can result in a cold-induced diuresis due to raised central venous pressure; this is prevented by moderate exercise in the cold.

The combination of exhaustion, hypoglycaemia, dehydration and hypothermia can represent a significant threat during exposure to the cold.

Clothing in the cold

Clothing in the cold should

- Prevent flushing of cold air/water beneath the garment, for example, have airtight/watertight seals
- Provide insulation by trapping a large volume of dry air close to the skin
- Enable adjustments in insulation to cater for times of increased/decreased metabolic heat production
- Be windproof
- Wick moisture away from the body for comfort
- Be vapour permeable to prevent condensation and accumulation of moisture under the clothing which, because of its high thermal capacity, will reduce clothing insulation

It is generally considered that when exercising in the cold, several layers of lighter clothing are better than one large bulky garment. The former approach enables clothing insulation to be adjusted to metabolic heat production more easily.

Strategies to maintain performance in the cold and avoid cold injury

Acclimatisation to cold

The most frequently reported acclimatisation to cold is characterised by a reduced shivering response (habituation), faster fall in deep body temperature ('hypothermic adaptation') and increased thermal comfort. This is typically seen in outdoor, long-distance swimmers at rest in cold water. The acclimation is specific to the deep body temperatures experienced during acclimatisation, with the habituated metabolic response returning to the response seen in unacclimated individuals when deep body temperature falls to lower levels than previously experienced.

Recent evidence seems to confirm earlier work that regular cold water swimmers (children and adults) develop a form of insulative acclimatisation to cold in which deep body temperature falls less with the same metabolic heat production when swimming in cold water.

The hazardous initial responses to immersion in cold water can be reduced by as much as 50% by as few as five 2-min immersions in cold water. A large part of this habituation appears to last for several months.

Hypothermia

Hypothermia exists when deep body temperature falls below 35 °C. Risk factors for hypothermia include the following:

- Cold air/water temperature
- Air/water movement: faster moving fluids increase convective heat loss
- Age: children cool faster than adults due to their lower levels of subcutaneous fat and higher surface area to mass ratio
- Body stature: tall thin individuals cool faster than short fat people
- Body morphology: body fat and unperfused muscle are good insulators
- Gender: females tend to have more subcutaneous fat than men
- Fitness: high fitness enables higher heat production
- Fatigue: exhaustion results in decreased heat production
- Nutritional state: hypoglycaemia attenuates shivering and accentuates cooling
- Intoxication: drug or alcohol depressant effects on metabolism
- Lack of appropriate clothing

Out of hospital treatment of hypothermia

- Lay casualty flat, give essential first aid, enquire about coexisting illness
- Prevent further heat loss (blankets/sleeping bag) – cover head, leave airway clear
- Insulate from the ground
- If possible provide shelter from the wind and rain
- Allow slow spontaneous rewarming to occur; rewarming too quickly can result in rewarming collapse
- Maintain close observation of pulse and respiration
- Obtain help as soon as possible and transport the casualty to hospital
- If breathing is absent, becomes obstructed or stops, standard expired air ventilation should be instituted
- Chest compression should only be started if:
  - There is not carotid pulse detectable after palpating for at least 1 min (the pulse is slow and weak in hypothermia) AND
  - Cardiac arrest is observed, or there is a reasonable possibility that a cardiac arrest occurred within the previous 2 h, AND
  - There is a reasonable expectation that effective cardiopulmonary resuscitation (CPR) can be provided continuously until the casualty reaches more advanced life support. This is likely to mean being within 2 h of a suitable hospital.
- The rates of expired air ventilation and chest compression should be the same as for normothermic casualties. Hypothermia may cause stiffness of the chest wall.

Cold injury

Cold injuries can be of the 'freezing' (frostbite) or non-freezing variety (NFCI).

Human tissue freezes at around −0.55 °C and depending on the rate of freezing intracellular crystals may form (rapid cooling) causing direct mechanical disruption of the tissues. The more common slow cooling and freezing results in predominantly extracellular water crystallisation that increases plasma and interstitial fluid osmotic pressure. The resulting osmotic outflow of intracellular fluid raises intracellular osmotic pressure and can cause damage to capillary walls. This, along with the local reduction in plasma volume, causes oedema, reduced local blood flow and encourages capillary sludging. These changes can produce thrombosis and a gangrenous extremity. The risk of frostbite is low above air temperatures of −7 °C, irrespective of wind speed, and becomes pronounced when ambient temperature is below −25 °C, even at low wind speeds.

NFCI is the term given to describe a condition that results from protracted exposure to low ambient thermal conditions, but in which freezing of tissues does not occur. Immobility, posture, dehydration, low fitness, inadequate nutrition, constricting footwear, fatigue, stress or anxiety, concurrent illness or injury can all increase the likelihood of NFCI.

Despite the fact that many sportspeople probably have at least moderate NFCI (especially those engaged in winter outdoor sports and water sports), the precise pathophysiology NFCI is poorly understood; the injury appears to be to the neuro-endothelio-muscular components of the walls of local blood vessels. Opinions vary as to whether the primary damage is vascular or neural in origin; or, whether the aetiology is primarily thermal, ischaemic, post-ischaemic reperfusion or hypoxic in origin. Recent evidence suggests that acute cold water immersion is associated with a loss of NO-dependent endothelial function and a defect in vascular smooth muscle contractility. Cold-induced activation of the Rho-kinase pathway may play a role in mediating cold-induced vascular injury, such as in the case of acute NFCI.

The chronic sequelae of mild-to-moderate cold injury are 'cold sensitivity' (protracted cold vasoconstriction following a cold stimulus) and hyperhidrosis (local increased sweating), both of which accentuate local cooling and thus increase future risk of cold injury. There appears to be variation in the susceptibility to NFCI between ethnic groups with African-Caribbean and Asian individuals being at greater risk.

Treatment

It is important to establish whether the dominant injury is freezing (FCI) or non-freezing (NFCI) in nature; this determines the preferred method of rewarming. In all cases, shelter should be sought, as casualties with cold injury are likely to be hypothermic they should be kept warm.

Frostbite

All cases of freezing injury should be thoroughly rewarmed by immersion of all the chilled part in stirred water at 38–42 °C. A topical anti-bacterial should also be diluted into the water bath. Rewarming should be delayed if there is a chance that refreezing may occur (Figure 14.3).

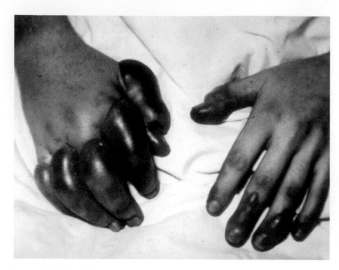

Figure 14.3 Frostbite

Thawing an FCI can be intensely painful. Conventional and narcotic analgesics should be provided as necessary. Continuing treatment for FCI is a twice daily, 30-min immersion of the affected part in a 38–42 °C whirlpool bath containing an appropriate anti-bacterial.

Non-freezing cold injury

In contrast to those with FCI, patients with NFCI should have their affected extremities rewarmed slowly, by exposure to warm air alone, and must not be immersed in warm water. The early period after rewarming can be very painful in NFCI, even in those without any obvious tissue damage. Amitriptyline (10–75 mg in a single dose at night) appears to assist with the treatment of pain following NFCI, and should be given as soon as pain is felt; it may cause drowsiness and hypertension (Figure 14.4).

With either form of injury, once rewarmed, the affected extremities should be treated by exposure to air and early mobilisation. Smoking should be prohibited.

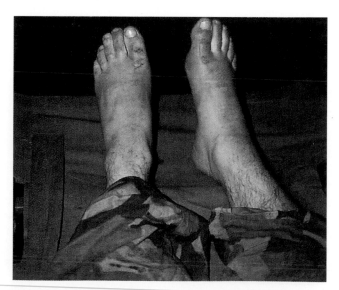

Figure 14.4 Non-freezing cold injury (pictures courtesy of Dr Frank Golden and the Cold Injuries Clinic, Institute of Naval Medicine, UK)

Ambient temperature (°C)										
	4	–1	–7	–12	–18	–23	–29	–34	–40	–46
Wind speed (mph)	**Wind chill (equivalent) temperature (°C)**									
5	2	–4	–12	–15	–21	–26	–32	–37	–43	–48
10	–1	–9	–15	–23	–29	–37	–34	–51	–57	–62
15	–4	–12	–21	–29	–34	–43	–51	–57	–65	–73
20	–7	–15	–23	–32	–37	–46	–54	–62	–71	–79
25	–9	–18	–26	–34	–43	–51	–59	–68	–76	–84
30	–12	–18	–29	–34	–46	–54	–62	–71	–79	–87
35	–12	–21	–29	–37	–46	–54	–62	–73	–82	–90
40	–12	–21	–29	–37	–48	–57	–65	–73	–82	–90
	Less danger			Increasing danger. Flesh may freeze within a minute			Great danger. Flesh may freeze within 30 seconds			

Figure 14.5 Wind chill chart: effect of increasing wind speed on degree of cooling at different ambient temperatures. Equivalent temperature is the environmental temperature that would have the same effect on bare skin in the absence of any wind (equivalent cooling power)

Assessing the risk of cold injuries

The cooling power of the environment is the result of air temperature and air movement or movement through air (e.g. as when skiing). These factors are combined into the Wind Chill Index, which illustrates the cooling effect of temperature and wind on bare skin and predicts the associated danger of cold injury (Figure 14.5).

Acknowledgements

Thanks to Dr Jo Corbett and Dr Heather Lunt, valued colleagues at the University of Portsmouth.

Further reading

Barwood, M.J., Davey, S., House, J.R. & Tipton, M.J. (2009) Post-exercise cooling techniques in hot, humid conditions. *European Journal of Applied Physiology*, **107**, 385–396. doi:10.1007/s00421-009-1135-1

Barwood, M., Datta, A., Thelwell, R. & Tipton, M. (2006) Breath-hold performance during cold water immersion: effects of psychological skills training. *Aviation Space Environmental Medicine*, **77** (**11**), 1136–1142.

Barwood, M., Thelwell, R. & Tipton, M. (2008) Psychological skills training improves exercise performance in the heat. *Medicine and Science in Exercise & Sport*, **40** (**2**), 398–396.

Bird, F., House, J., Lunt, H. & Tipton, M.J. (2012) *The Physiological and Subjective Responses to Repeated Cold Water Immersion in a Group of 10–12 Year Olds*. FINA Conference Istanbul, Turkey.

Corbett, J., Barwood, M.J., Lunt, H.C., Milner, A. & Tipton, M.J. (2011) Water immersion as a recovery aid from intermittent shuttle running exercise. *European Journal of Sport Science*, **12** (**6**): 509–14.

Dugas, J. (2011) Ice slurry ingestion increase running time in the heat. *Clinical Journal of Sport Medicine*, **21** (**6**), 541–542. doi:10.1097/01.jsm.0000407930.13102.42

Francis, TJR. & Oakley, EHN. Cold injury. Chapter 23, pages 353–370 *A Textbook of Vascular Medicine*, ed. JE Tooke & GDO Lowe. Arnold, London. 1996.

Golden FS, Hampton IF, Smith D. Lean long distance swimmers. *Journal of the Royal Naval Medical Service* 1980; Spring **66** (**1**), 26–30.

Golden, F.S. & Tipton, M.J. (2002) *Essentials of Sea Survival*. Human Kinetics, Champaign, IL, US.

Heled Y, Peled A, Yanovich R, Shargal E, Pilz-Burstein R, Epstein Y, Moran DS. Heat acclimation and performance in hypoxic conditions. *Aviation, Space, and Environmental Medicine* 2012; July, **83** (**7**), 649–653.

Lind, A.R. (1963) A physiological criterion for setting thermal environmental limits for everyday work. *Journal of Applied Physiology*, **18** (**1**), 51–56.

Lorenzo, S., Halliwill, J.R., Sawka, M.N. & Minson, C.T. (2010) Heat acclimation improves exercise performance. *Journal of Applied Physiology*, **109**, 1140–1147. doi:10.1152/japplphysiol.00495.2010

Lunt, H.C., Barwood, M.J., Corbett, J. & Tipton, M.J. (2010) "Cross-adaptation": habituation to short repeated cold-water immersions affects the response to acute hypoxia in humans. *Journal of Physiology*, **588** (**18**), 3605–3613.

Milledge, J.S. (1998) Altitude. In: Harries, M., Williams, C., Stanish, W.D. & Micheli, L.J. (eds), *Oxford Textbook of Sports Medicine*, 2nd edn. Oxford University Press, Oxford.

Muggeridge, D.J., Howe, C.C., Spendiff, O., Pedlar, C., James, P.E. & Easton, C. (2014) A Single Dose of Beetroot Juice Enhances Cycling Performance in Simulated Altitude. *Medicine and Science in Sports and Exercise*, **46** (**1**), 143–150.

Rowell, L.B. *et al.* (1966) Reductions in cardiac output, central blood volume, and stroke volume with thermal stress in normal men during exercise. *The Journal of Clinical Investigation*, **45**, 1801–1816.

Siegel, R., Mate, J., Brearley, M.B., Watson, G., Nosaka, K. & Laursen, P.B. (2010) Ice slurry ingestion increases core temperature capacity and running time in the heat. *Medicine and Science in Sports and Exercise*, **42** (**4**), 717–725.

Stephens JP, Laight DW, Golden FStC, Tipton MJ. Damage to vascular endothelium and smooth muscle contribute to the development of non-freezing cold injury in the rat tail vascular bed *in vitro*. Proceedings of the ICEE meeting Boston 2009.

Tipton, M.J. (2013) Sudden cardiac death during open water swimming. *Tipton MJ. Br J Sports Med*. 2014 Aug; **48** (**15**): 1134–5.

Tipton, M., Wakabayashi, H., Barwood, M., Eglin, C., Mekjavic, I. & Taylor, N. (2013) Habituation of the metabolic and ventilatory responses to cold-water immersion in humans. *Journal of Thermal Biology*, **38** (**1**), 24–31. ISSN 0306-4565. IF 1.392

White, G.E. & Wells, G.D. (2013) Cold-water immersion and other forms of cryotherapy: physiological changes potentially affecting recovery from high-intensity exercise. *Extreme Physiology & Medicine*, **2**, 26. doi:10.1186/2046-7648-2-26

Youngman E, Howe C, Moir H. The effects of alti-vit on exercise performance at altitude. *British Journal of Sports Medicine* 2013; Nov, **47** (**17**), e4. doi:10.1136/bjsports-2013-093073.22.

CHAPTER 15

Diving Medicine

Peter T. Wilmshurst

University Hospital of North Midlands, Stoke-on-Trent, UK

OVERVIEW

In this chapter we describe diving medicine. After studying this chapter, the reader will know

- The effects of immersion
- The effects of pressure
- Breath-hold diving
- SCUBA diving
- Barotrauma and decompression illness

Introduction

There are two types of recreational diving. A breath-hold dive, often using mask, fins and snorkel, is of short duration. Scuba diving, using self-contained underwater breathing apparatus, considerably increases the dive duration. The essential equipment for scuba divers is the demand valve, which delivers gas to the diver's lungs at ambient pressure and makes it possible to breathe despite the high ambient pressures underwater (Figure 15.1).

Competitive sports undertaken by breath-hold divers include underwater hockey in a swimming pool, and depth and endurance record attempts. Underwater orienteering is a competitive sport for scuba divers.

Divers are exposed to dangers from immersion, from the pressure underwater and from a hostile environment, including trauma and venomous marine animals.

Effects of immersion

Cooling

All seas are cooler than body temperature. Water has a thermal capacity and thermal conductivity, respectively, about 3000 and 32 times greater than air. So divers are cooled quickly during immersion, in all but tropical waters, unless they have adequate thermal insulation from a wet suit or a dry suit. Even with thermal insulation, hypothermia can occur with prolonged immersion.

ABC of Sports and Exercise Medicine, Fourth Edition.
Edited by Gregory P. Whyte, Mike Loosemore and Clyde Williams.
© 2015 John Wiley & Sons, Ltd. Published 2015 by John Wiley & Sons, Ltd.

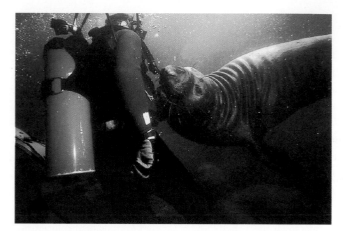

Figure 15.1 A dive to 30 m for 20 min puts the scuba diver at risk of nitrogen narcosis and decompression illness. The elephant seal can dive to 1 km for an hour without risk of either condition

Hydrostatic effects

Immersion increases venous return by the hydraulic effect of water pressure on the limbs. In warm water, intrathoracic blood volume increases by up to 700 ml, which increases right atrial pressures by 18 mm Hg, cardiac output by over 30% and blood pressure slightly. These effects may be potentiated by peripheral vasoconstriction from cooling. In some individuals, the combined effects are sufficient to cause cardiac decompensation and immersion pulmonary oedema (Figure 15.2). The increased central blood volume causes natriuresis and diuresis. During prolonged immersion, the resulting reduction in plasma volume is so great that, when the diver is rescued and removed from the water and hydrostatic support of venous return is removed, hypovolaemic shock and sometimes death occur. To minimise this, casualties, who have had prolonged immersion, should be lifted from the water with the body horizontal, rather than with legs dependent.

Effects of pressure

At sea level atmospheric pressure is 1 bar absolute (1 standard atmosphere = 101 kPa = 1.013 bars). For each 10 m, a diver descends the pressure increases by 1 bar and the volume of gas in a compressible container, such as a breath-hold diver's lungs, is reduced in proportion to the increase in pressure.

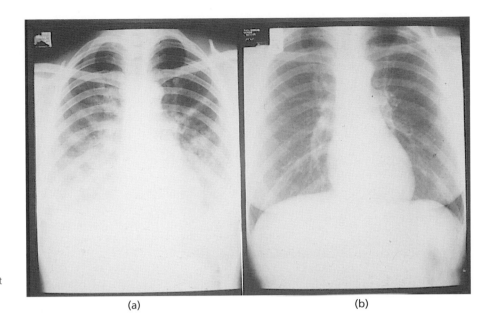

(a)   (b)

Figure 15.2 Chest X-ray showing immersion pulmonary oedema (a) that resolved quickly without treatment after the diver was removed from the water (b)

Dry air is approximately 21% oxygen, 78% nitrogen and 1% other gases. The partial pressures of oxygen at any depth will be 21% of the total pressure exerted by the air and the partial pressure of nitrogen will be 78% of total pressure. Gases dissolve in a liquid with which they are in contact. Nitrogen is soluble in fat, and at sea level we have several litres dissolved in our tissues. If the partial pressure of nitrogen is doubled (by breathing air at 10 m depth) for long enough so that equilibration occurs, we will contain twice as many dissolved nitrogen molecules as at sea level.

Doubling the inspired partial pressure of oxygen, doubles the amount of oxygen dissolved in tissues but it does not double the amount of oxygen in the body because most of our oxygen content is bound to oxygen carrying pigments. The haemoglobin in arterial blood is virtually saturated at an inspired partial pressure of oxygen (P_iO_2) of 21 kPa. So increasing the partial pressure of oxygen has little effect on the amount of oxygen bound to haemoglobin.

Breath-hold diving

During a breath-hold, the oxygen content of tissues decreases, but the breath-hold is broken in a healthy person because of carbon dioxide production and resulting acidosis, which stimulates the respiratory centre. The breath-hold can be extended by hyperventilation before the breath-hold. Hyperventilation has little effect on oxygen content of the body, but it eliminates carbon dioxide, so that the breath-hold starts with a higher cerebrospinal fluid pH. Hyperventilation does not alter the rates of oxygen consumption or carbon dioxide production, but the lower initial carbon dioxide content means that hypoxia triggers respiration long before the pH of cerebrospinal fluid falls enough to do so.

Hyperventilation before diving will enables breath-hold divers to stay down longer but it is dangerous. The diver starts with a low carbon dioxide content and a normal oxygen tension. During descent to, say, 30 m, the pressure increases fourfold, compressing the lungs to one-quarter their volume at the surface. The partial pressures of oxygen and nitrogen in the alveoli increase fourfold and produce corresponding increases in arterial and tissue gas tensions. During the dive, oxygen is consumed and carbon dioxide is produced. Because of the prior hyperventilation, the diver does not feel the need to breathe until the arterial oxygen tension falls enough to stimulate the respiratory centre and the diver ascends. During the ascent, hydrostatic pressure is reduced fourfold with a fourfold reduction of the oxygen tensions in alveolar gas, arterial blood and tissues. The rapidly falling cerebral oxygen tension may be insufficient for consciousness to be maintained and the diver could drown during the ascent.

The danger of hyperventilation applies to all breath-hold divers, including people swimming lengths underwater in swimming pools. The reduction in oxygen tension when coming to the surface from the bottom of a 2 m deep pool can be enough to cause unconsciousness.

Scuba diving

Air

The cheapest gas to use for scuba diving is air. Nitrogen is not inert at the high partial pressures achieved when breathing air at depth. It affects cell membranes to cause nitrogen narcosis. Mild impairment of intellectual function may occur at 30 m, with progressive impairment as the diver descends and unconsciousness at depths near 100 m.

The nitrogen that dissolves in the tissues at depth also needs to be liberated on ascent or decompression. Because nitrogen is highly soluble, a large volume of gas may be involved (Figure 15.3). If the rate of decompression (ascent) is too rapid, large amounts of bubbles are liberated from the supersaturated tissues. For some deep or long dives, decompression stops are performed to permit gas liberation at a safe rate without excessive bubble formation before continuing the ascent. The release of small amounts of bubbles is common after innocuous dives, but excess bubbles or bubbles in the wrong place cause decompression illness.

Nitrogen is also a relatively dense gas, which makes the work of breathing at 30 m twice as great as at the surface.

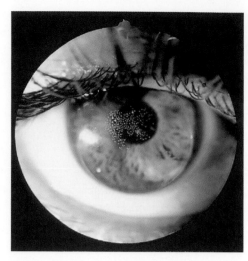

Figure 15.3 Bubbles formed during decompression may be visible in tear fluid beneath a contact lens

Oxygen

One way to deal with the difficulties with nitrogen is to breathe 100% oxygen using a re-breathing system. The diver breathes into and out of a bellows-like counter-lung with the oxygen used being topped up from a cylinder of gas and chemical absorption of carbon dioxide produced. Divers breathing pure oxygen need to carry much smaller amounts of gas, but there are problems. An inefficient carbon dioxide absorber may cause carbon dioxide toxicity and hence incapacity and drowning. If water enters the carbon dioxide absorber, the diver may inhale a caustic cocktail causing severe lung injury. At a P_iO_2 greater than 160 kPa, acute oxygen toxicity can cause convulsions without warning. A convulsion underwater is usually fatal. The higher the P_iO_2, the greater is the risk. When breathing air, containing 21% oxygen, there is a risk of acute oxygen toxicity at depths greater than 66 m, but when breathing 100% oxygen, there is a risk of convulsion at only 6 m.

Nitrox

Amateur divers often breathe a nitrogen–oxygen (nitrox) mixture with the oxygen percentage higher than air. For example, nitrox 40 consists of 40% oxygen and 60% nitrogen. The reduced nitrogen content compared with air increases the dive duration with a low risk of decompression illness on surfacing. The trade-off is that there is a risk of convulsion from acute oxygen toxicity if the diver descends too deep. Computerised re-breathers are increasingly used to supply amateur divers with nitrox mixtures that vary according to the depth of the dive.

Mixed gas diving

Deeper than 66 m, the gas mixture should contain a lower concentration of oxygen than 21% to avoid the risk of acute oxygen toxicity. The general rule is to try to achieve a gas mixture giving a P_iO_2 of about 130 kPa. However, the reduction cannot be achieved by addition of nitrogen because that would increase the risk of nitrogen narcosis and decompression illness. Commonly, helium is used as a component of the breathing gas for deep dives. Helium molecules

are small, so that the work of breathing is low even at great depths. It is relatively insoluble in lipids, minimising bubble liberation on decompression. Unfortunately, helium is expensive and it has a high thermal conductivity, which increases heat loss. Thus, hypothermia is a serious possibility on deep dives. Amateur deep divers use various mixtures of oxygen, nitrogen and helium called trimix. Different mixtures will be used at different stages of descent and ascent.

Barotrauma

The gas contained within body cavities (middles ear, sinuses and lungs) will be compressed as a breath-hold diver descends. Pain as the eardrum is pushed inwards may limit the depth achieved in a breath-hold dive. If the descent continues the eardrum may rupture inwards, the round or oval window may rupture outwards or there may be haemorrhage into the middle ear.

Scuba divers perform manoeuvres to equalise pressures during descent to prevent barotrauma occurring, but equalisation may be prevented if the Eustachian tube or the mouth of a sinus is blocked. Barotrauma to ears and sinuses are frequent injuries of divers. A respiratory tract infection will increase the risk of barotrauma.

Scuba divers may also experience pulmonary barotrauma on ascent, if they make a rapid ascent without exhaling adequately or have lung disease causing gas trapping. Gas expands as pressure is reduced and failure to equalise pressure can cause lung rupture. For example, during ascent from a dive to 30 m, the volume of gas in a bulla will increase fourfold as ambient pressure is reduced if the bulla is unable to empty adequately, and it will burst causing local lung damage, pneumothorax, surgical emphysema or gas embolism. In divers, the most common is gas embolism when gas invades the pulmonary veins and passes to the systemic circulation. Usually bubbles pass up the carotid arteries to cause neurological injury. If a pneumothorax occurs during ascent, the gas in the pleural space will expand according to Boyle's law as pressure is reduced causing a tension pneumothorax.

Decompression illness

After many innocuous dives, venous bubbles are formed. Most bubbles are filtered in the pulmonary capillaries and do not reach the systemic circulation. In individuals with a persistent foramen ovale or other right-to-left shunt, there can be paradoxical gas embolism of bubbles with venous bubbles evading the pulmonary filter to cause neurological effects. After provocative dives so many bubbles may be liberated that the pulmonary filter is overwhelmed. Other features of decompression illness are cardio-respiratory symptoms, joint pain and skin involvement (Figures 15.4 and Table 15.1). Treatment of decompression illness is with hyperbaric oxygen in a compression chamber (Figure 15.5).

Amateur scuba diving

Deaths and serious illness when diving occur when divers fail to follow accepted safety precautions, equipment fails or disease placed the diver at risk. Clubs and commercial schools train sport divers through theory and pool training to progressively more challenging and deeper open water dives.

Table 15.1 Causes of decompression illness

	Right-to-left shunt permitting paradoxical gas embolism	Lung disease causing pulmonary barotrauma	Provocative dive profile (missed decompression stops or rapid ascent)
Neurological	Over half the cases	About a quarter of cases	Nearly a quarter of cases
Cardiorespiratory	About half the cases	About a quarter of cases	About a quarter of cases
Skin	About three quarters of cases	0	About a quarter of cases
Joint	Few if any cases	0	Almost all cases

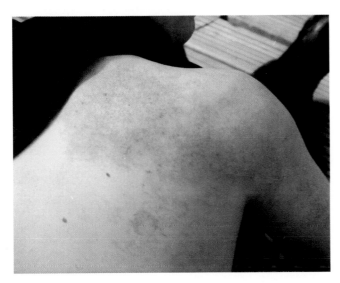

Figure 15.4 Skin bends (cutaneous decompression illness) are typically situated on the trunk and have a mottled or marbled red, blue and purple appearance. Most are the result of paradoxical gas embolism across a shunt, but some are the result of an unsafe dive profile

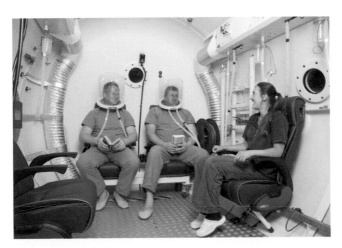

Figure 15.5 A demonstration of the arrangements for treating patients in a compression chamber. Source: DDRC Healthcare

Before someone is allowed to start diving and periodically when diving, they have to complete a medical questionnaire to ensure freedom from diseases that might predispose to incapacity in the water or to diving-related illnesses. The responses determine whether divers need examination by an approved diving medical referee.

Lung diseases that impair exercise capacity or predispose to pulmonary barotrauma on ascent are contraindications to diving.

Usually people with mild asthma are fit to dive but smokers may not be.

People are advised not to dive if they have a condition that might cause incapacity in the water (e.g. epilepsy and serious cardiac diseases) or predispose to diving-related diseases. Hypertension predisposes to diving induced pulmonary oedema. Intracardiac shunts predispose to decompression illness. Pacemakers contain gas and are compressed by the pressure underwater. This can cause the pacemaker to fail at depth. Some medications have unanticipated effects in divers because hyperbaric conditions may modify their actions. There are schemes that allow some disabled individuals to scuba dive.

Summary

Breath-hold diving and scuba diving expose divers to the effects of immersion, including the risk of hypothermia and circulatory consequences of immersion. The latter include increased central blood volume that can contribute to immersion pulmonary oedema. Hyperventilation before a breath-hold dive may cause loss of consciousness on ascent. High partial pressures of oxygen at depth can cause acute oxygen toxicity, which results in convulsions. The raised partial pressures of nitrogen when diving may cause nitrogen narcosis underwater and decompression illness on ascent. Decompression illness can occur after theoretically safe dives particularly when a right-to-left shunt allows venous bubbles to bypass the lung filter. Pulmonary barotrauma can result from a rapid ascent or during a normal ascent in divers with some lung diseases.

Summary

- Breath-hold diving and scuba divers are exposed to the effects of immersion, including the risk of hypothermia.
- Immersion increases central blood volume and can cause pulmonary oedema.
- Hyperventilation before a breath-hold dive may cause loss of consciousness on ascent.
- High partial pressures of oxygen at depth can cause convulsions.
- The raised partial pressures of nitrogen when diving may cause nitrogen narcosis and decompression illness on ascent.
- Decompression illness can occur after theoretically safe dives particularly when a right-to-left shunt allows venous bubbles to bypass the lung filter.
- Pulmonary barotrauma can result from a rapid ascent or during a normal ascent in divers with lung disease.

Further reading

Sport diving. The British Sub-Aqua Club Diving Manual. British Sub-Aqua Club, Telford's Quay, Ellesmere Port, Cheshire L65 4FY.

Edmonds, C., Lowry, C., Pennefather, J. & Walker, R. (2002) *Diving and Sub-aquatic Medicine*, 4th edn. Hodder Headline Group, London.

Medical standards for divers

U.K. Sport Diving Medical Committee website: www.uksdmc.co.uk

British Thoracic Society guideline on respiratory aspects of fitness for diving. *Thorax* 2003, **58**, 3–13.

Governing bodies for amateur scuba diving in the United Kingdom

British Sub-Aqua Club: www.bsac.com
Scottish Sub-Aqua Club: www.scotsac.com

CHAPTER 16

Altitude Medicine

Sundeep Dhillon

Centre for Aviation Space & Extreme Environment Medicine, University College London, London, UK

OVERVIEW

This chapter describes the physiological and medical challenges of altitude.

After studying this chapter, the reader will be able to

- Describe the physiological effects of high altitude and acclimatisation
- Outline the recognition, management and prevention of the most important high-altitude illnesses:
  - Acute Mountain Sickness (AMS)
  - High-Altitude Cerebral Oedema (HACE)
  - High-Altitude Pulmonary Oedema (HAPE)
- Understand the challenges for athletes competing at high altitude
- Discuss training at altitude to improve athletic performance at sea level

---

Box 16.1 **Problems associated with increasing altitude**

- Reduced barometric pressure – at Everest Base Camp (5300 m), there is approximately half of the oxygen available compared with sea level. On the summit (8848 m), it falls to one-third. It is lower in winter and at higher latitudes.
- Cold – temperature decreases by approximately 1 °C for every 150 m gain in altitude. Any wind on exposed skin increases the risk of frostbite from wind-chill.
- Reduced humidity – need to increase fluid intake, especially as thirst suppressed at altitude.
- Ozone – irritates mucous membranes and can cause bronchoconstriction and shortness of breath.
- Increased ultraviolet radiation – increases by 10–12% for every 1000 m altitude gain, so there is twice as much radiation at 4000 m compared with sea level increasing risk of sunburn, snow-blindness and skin cancer.

Drug dosages are given as a guide only and should be checked. Medicines should only be used under supervision of an appropriate and competent medical authority.

Introduction

We evolved at sea level and with the exception of the high-altitude populations of Central Asia and South America (who have adapted over many generations to the decreased atmospheric oxygen) are poorly suited to high altitude. The most significant problem is hypobaric hypoxia (low oxygen levels as a result of a reduced barometric pressure), but other factors make the high-altitude environment physiologically challenging (Box 16.1). Nevertheless, over 140 million people live at altitudes above 2500 m with a similar number of lowlanders visiting these altitudes annually.

What is high altitude?

There is no universally accepted definition of high altitude, but it is useful to consider the physiological effects on the body (Box 16.2). There is considerable individual variation with some individuals

suffering with acute exposure to 1500–2000 m. Most people will suffer to a greater or lesser degree with rapid ascent above 2500 m (the approximate altitude to which a commercial airplane is pressurised). The majority of altitude illness occurs between 2500 and 3500 m due to the large number of people ascending rapidly to these altitudes, mainly for recreational purposes.

Acclimatisation

Acute exposure to the summit of Mt Everest (8848 m) would result in loss of consciousness within a few minutes, followed rapidly by death. A few people have, however, managed to climb Everest without the use of supplemental oxygen. This is only possible due to a number of physiological adaptations (acclimatisation), which partially compensates for the decreased oxygen. Increases in heart rate and respiratory rate are accompanied by a decrease in exercise capacity (maximum heart rate falls combined with low-Hb oxygen saturation). Haemoglobin (Hb) increases along with a raft of other biochemical adjustments, which aim to improve oxygen delivery and utilisation. Lean muscle mass is lost disproportionately to fat. The microcirculation becomes increasingly sluggish and despite compensatory mitochondrial adjustments, performance at altitude decreases and does not return to sea level values, even with the administration of 100% oxygen.

ABC of Sports and Exercise Medicine, Fourth Edition.
Edited by Gregory P. Whyte, Mike Loosemore and Clyde Williams.
© 2015 John Wiley & Sons, Ltd. Published 2015 by John Wiley & Sons, Ltd.

Box 16.2 Description of high altitudes according to physiological effects

Description	Altitude (m)	Physiological effects
Low altitude	< 1500	No effect on healthy individuals
Intermediate altitude	1500–2500	Arterial oxygen saturation (SaO_2) remains above 90% – altitude illness possible
High altitude	2500–3500	Altitude illness common with rapid ascent above 2500 m
Very high altitude	3500–5800	(SaO_2) falls below 90%, especially with exertion/exercise. Altitude illness is common even with gradual ascent
Extreme altitude	> 5800	Limit of permanent human habitation, progressive deterioration with increased length of stay eventually outstrips acclimatisation, marked difficulty at rest

Source: Data from Pollard and Murdoch, *The High Altitude Medicine Handbook*

Unlike adaptation, where favourable characteristics are genetically selected over many generations, the effects of acclimatisation are lost exponentially over 2–3 weeks following descent to low altitudes. The rate of acclimatisation varies between individuals with most changes occurring within 1–20 days. There is no sea-level predictive test of performance at altitude, although previous experience is a reasonable guide. Age, gender and physical fitness have no relationship to development of altitude illnesses.

High-altitude illnesses

Ascending to high altitude too rapidly can result in a range of disorders which may be life threatening. They are best prevented using a gentle ascent profile allowing adequate time to acclimatise. Some people will be susceptible to the effects of high altitude even with an extremely conservative ascent profile. Awareness, early recognition and prompt management of high-altitude illnesses are vital for both team physicians, support staff and athletes.

Acute mountain sickness (AMS)

Case study

You are the team doctor to a charity expedition to Mt. Kilimanjaro (5895 m) in Tanzania – the highest mountain in Africa. Having ascended from the park gate (1640 m) to Machame Camp (3000 m) the previous day, several members of your group make slow progress to Shira camp (3840 m) taking 9 h (most of the group did it in 4–6 h). On arrival they are exhausted and go straight to sleep as they do not feel hungry. Two of them wake you at 0200 hours with the worst headaches they have ever had, which have not responded to paracetamol.

Kilimanjaro is the highest freestanding mountain in the world and a popular destination for charity climbs. The rate of ascent on Kilimanjaro far exceeds any recommended guidelines, and there is considerable under-reported altitude-related morbidity. Costs are proportional to the number of days spent on the mountain so the fastest routes are the cheapest and most popular. Forty-five percentage of the approximately 40,000 people attempting Kilimanjaro every year use the Machame route. It is possible to go from the Park Gate at 1640 m to the summit in 4–5 days, a gain of 4255 m (Box 16.3). Summit success rates are between 45 and 60%. One hundred and ninety out of one hundred and ninety-eight trekkers (96%) on the Caudwell Xtreme Everest expedition in 2007 reached Everest Base Camp in 11 days, an altitude gain of 4000 m (Box 16.4).

The rate of ascent is probably the most important modifiable factor in preventing high-altitude illness. In Nepal, 50% of trekkers getting to 4000 m in 5 days suffered from AMS compared with 84% of those who flew directly to 3860 m. Above 3000 m, the recommendation is to ascend no more than 300–500 m per day with a rest day every 3–4 days. This may be infuriatingly slow for some members of the team, but provides an opportunity for most people to acclimatise. Like most guidelines, this strategy does not guarantee that everyone will be protected, and ascent profiles should be modified to accommodate the slowest member of the group.

The symptoms of AMS are headache, nausea, vomiting, lethargy, fatigue, loss of appetite and poor sleep. None are specific and other conditions such as dehydration, hypothermia, hypoglycaemia, exhaustion and viral infections are also common and may occur concurrently. AMS must be excluded in the mountains,

Box 16.3 Poor ascent profile for the Machame route on Kilimanjaro

Altitude (m)	Location	Height gain (m)
1640	Park gate	
3000	Machame	1360
3840	Shira	840
3900	Barranco	60
4600	Barafu	700
5895	Uhuru – summit	1295
	Total height gain	4255
	Ascent rate metre per day	851
	Rest days	0

Box 16.4 **Good ascent profile for trekking to Everest Base Camp**

Altitude (m)	Location	Height gain (m)
1300	Kathmandu	
2835	Lukla/Monjo	1535
3440	Namche Bazaar	605
3440	Namche Bazaar	0
3440	Namche Bazaar	0
3700	Debouche	260
4270	Pheriche	570
4270	Pheriche	0
4270	Pheriche	0
4840	Lobuje	570
5220	Gorak Shep	380
5380	Everest Base Camp	160
	Total height gain	4080
	Ascent rate metre per day	371
	Rest days	4

particularly if there has been a recent height gain. The mechanism is poorly understood, but thought to involve increased microvascular permeability, exacerbated by increased cerebral venous pressure. Failure of the blood–brain barrier is compounded by cytotoxic inflammatory mediators.

Treatment involves avoiding any further ascent until symptoms have resolved, simple painkillers (paracetamol or ibuprofen) for headache and acetazolamide (250 mg twice daily). With severe AMS (or if the symptoms do not improve with the above) dexamethasone 4 mg every 6 h may be used along with supplemental oxygen.

Acetazolamide 125 mg twice daily is effective as a prophylaxis to reduce the incidence of AMS in susceptible individuals, or when a large height gain is unavoidable. It is most effective if taken a few days before going to altitude.

Case study conclusion

The Kilimanjaro trekkers had AMS and were treated with a combination of paracetamol and acetazolamide. Following 2 days resting at the same altitude, the groups were able to continue and all successfully reached the summit.

Porters in many mountain regions such as the Himalaya and East Africa are not high-altitude natives and are just as prone to altitude sickness as Western lowlanders – in many cases more so as they are working considerably harder carrying supplies. Any responsible doctor will ensure that expedition porters are well equipped for the conditions, insured against medical and evacuation costs, aware of the dangers of altitude and have free access to the expedition doctor without prejudice to their income.

High-altitude cerebral oedema (HACE)

Case study

On 21 May 2007, climbers descending from the summit of Mt Everest found an unconscious Nepalese climber at around 8500 m. She was taken down to the South Col (7950 m) where doctors from the Caudwell Xtreme Everest expedition treated her for frostbite and cerebral oedema and coordinated her evacuation to Kathmandu. She made a full recovery and successfully summited Everest the following year.

HACE is a life-threatening form of altitude illness. Fortunately, it is rare affecting around 1–2% of people ascending to > 4500 m. It is usually preceded by AMS, but can occur without warning. The cardinal feature is ataxia (best tested by heel–toe walking with the eyes closed). HACE is often accompanied by strange and inappropriate behaviour (also seen in hypothermia that may co-exist) and loss of survival instincts (such as removing gloves). Almost any neurological sign and symptom may be seen including strokes, but the most common are confusion, disorientation, hallucinations and an inability to pass urine. If untreated, it can rapidly lead to unconsciousness, coma and death. HACE is at the opposite end of the same spectrum of disease from AMS (AMS is mild HACE).

The main treatment is immediate descent. Dexamethasone 8 mg is given immediately followed by 4 mg every 6 h. Supplemental oxygen should be given if available. A portable hyperbaric chamber may also be beneficial and should be considered by all teams ascending to very high/extreme altitudes. Other altitude illnesses commonly occur along with HACE, and both acetazolamide and nifedipine may be considered.

High-altitude pulmonary oedema (HAPE)

Case study

On descending from the summit of Aconcagua in Argentina (6962 m), a young female climber became increasingly tired and breathless. On arriving back at Camp 2 (5700 m), she began to cough up blood-stained sputum and complained of pain in her chest. On examination at rest, she was found to have a respiratory rate of 44 breaths per minutes, a heart rate of 142 beats per minutes and an arterial oxygen saturation of 65%. A diagnosis of HAPE was made, and 30 mg of slow release (SR) nifedipine was given. With her friends carrying her equipment, she was able to descend to Base Camp (4200 m). The following morning, she was evacuated by helicopter to the local hospital. After 2 days of treatment, she was given the 'all clear' and discharged home.

The incidence of HAPE may be 10% with rapid ascents to > 4500 m, but 1–2% is more likely with a sensible ascent profile. Subclinical HAPE is thought to be present in many people at altitude contributing to the reduced SaO_2. HAPE typically occurs on the second night after ascending to high altitude and is more common following a viral upper respiratory tract infection. It may be preceded by AMS and is manifested by shortness of breath, initially on exertion (out of proportion to the activity) and then as the disease progresses to dyspnoea at rest. This is often exacerbated at night by lying down and may be accompanied by a wet, bubbly productive cough with blood in the sputum (pink or red stained). Chest pain and headache occur in around two-thirds of cases. A dry cough is common at altitude due to the dry air – if there are no other symptoms, this is unlikely to be related to HAPE. An increased heart rate and respiratory rate are usually found even at rest. Patent foramen ovale increases the risk of HAPE by a factor of 4. Individuals with underlying respiratory tract infections are at increased risk as are those who are particularly energetic on arrival at altitude, who should be encouraged to minimise exertion.

The pathophysiology is massively increased pulmonary arterial pressure and stress failure of pulmonary capillaries. ECG findings range from tachycardia to peaked p waves (*p pulmonale*), right-axis deviation, inverted T waves and occasionally ST segment elevation. Individuals who have developed HAPE remain susceptible to further episodes (possibly for life) even after recovering from the initial insult.

Treatment is immediate descent and nifedipine SR 60 mg is given daily in two to three doses. Supplemental oxygen and a portable hyperbaric chamber may be used if available. Antibiotics should be considered if there is any suggestion of chest infection.

People who have suffered an episode of HAPE remain susceptible to further episodes of HAPE (usually around the same altitude as the original episode). Further ascent is inadvisable, but if unavoidable nifedipine may be used prophylactically. There is some evidence that inhaled salmeterol (125 µg twice daily) may also be effective. Prophylaxis against HAPE should not be a substitute for graded ascent.

Box 16.6 **Other problems of high altitude**

- Gastrointestinal upset – may be due to contaminated water or snow (hidden by fresh snow), poor hygiene in the group or alluvial deposits in glacial melt water.
- Sleep – respiratory drive at altitude is dependent on carbon dioxide production rather than hypoxia. The respiratory centre is depressed when sleeping and periodic breathing with alternating hypo- and hyperventilation is common. Irregular shallow breathing and apnoeic pauses (of up to 30 s) result in fitful hypoxic sleep patterns similar to obstructive sleep apnoea. Acetazolamide 125 mg at night may be used to treat periodic breathing.
- Cough – almost universal with increasing stay at altitude. Poorly understood (involves hypoxia and hyperventilation of cold dry air) and hard to treat. May be severe enough to disrupt sleep and even fracture ribs.
- Central nervous system – almost any pathology ranging from migraines and focal nerve palsies through to strokes can present at altitude in otherwise healthy individuals.
- Retinal haemorrhages – present in up to 50% of trekkers at Everest Base Camp (5300 m) and 90% of climbers above 7600 m. Multiple flame-shaped haemorrhages are adjacent to blood vessels and asymptomatic unless there is macular involvement. Usually resolve spontaneously over weeks at sea level. If vision loss is due to haemorrhage it is usually painless, but demands evacuation to low-altitude definitive care.
- Corneal thickening – may cause blurring or loss of vision in people who have undergone refractive surgery (RK and LASIK). PRK seems to be least affected by high altitude.
- Thromboembolic disease – increasing altitude may increase blood viscosity and increase the risk of thromboembolic events, particularly in those with an underlying risk factors for coagulopathy.

Box 16.5 **Summary of medical management of altitude–related disorders**

Medication	Indication	Adult dose	Route
Acetazolamide	Prevention of AMS and HACE	125 mg every 12 h	Oral
	Treatment of AMS	250 mg every 12 h	Oral
Dexamethasone	Prevention of AMS and HACE	2 mg every 6 h or 4 mg every 12 h	Oral
	Treatment of AMS	4 mg every 6 h	Oral IV IM
	Treatment of HACE	8 mg stat *followed by* 4 mg every 6 h	Oral IV IM
Nifedipine	Prevention and treatment of HAPE	60 mg SR daily (30 mg SR twice daily or 20 mg SR every 8 h)	Oral

Source: Adapted from Luks *et al.* (2010) "Wilderness Medical Society Consensus Guidelines for the Prevention and Treatment of Acute Altitude Illness". Reproduced with permission from Elsevier

Descending to a lower altitude is the most effective and definitive treatment for all forms of altitude illness

The medical management of common altitude-related disorders is summarised in Box 16.5. A multitude of other problems may be associated with high altitude (Box 16.6).

The athlete at altitude

The reduced air density at high altitude favours sprint events, but the lower oxygen levels reduce VO_{2max} (by 7.7% for every 1000 m of altitude) resulting in slower times for endurance events. The 1968 Mexico Games held in Mexico (2250 m) resulted in records being set in 200 m, 400 m and the long jump. VO_{2max} at this altitude is 84% of sea level values, which is manifested by an increase in 800 m times by around 2.6% rising to 14.9% for 10,000 m. There appears to be a threshold altitude above 1500 m with marathon times increasing between 1.5 and 3.5% for every 300 m of altitude gained above 1500 m. Around half of endurance athletes desaturate with maximal exercise at sea level and this is compounded with increasing altitude.

Acclimatisation to altitude increases oxygen delivery to tissues, mainly through polycythemia, but this may be negated by increases in plasma viscosity and microcirculatory derangement.

Overall, the maximum intensity of training is reduced and detraining may occur. This paradox means that athletes intending to compete at altitude should allow adequate time to acclimatise, but balance this against not being able to train to sea-level norms. Around 21 days is required for optimal acclimatisation.

A variety of training regimes at altitude have been devised using both natural hypobaric hypoxia and normobaric hypoxia (hypoxic chambers and tents); however, the results vary and the precise prescription and duration of hypoxia has not been conclusively established. Readers are referred to the *BASES Expert Statement on Human Performance in Hypoxia Inducing Environments* for a more detailed discussion of this subject.

Athletes and team physicians should consult the World Anti-Doping Agency (WADA). Both acetazolamide and dexamethasone are classified as performance enhancing drugs and are on the WADA prohibited list. Athletes are prohibited from 'Artificially enhancing the uptake, transport or delivery of oxygen'.

Athletes should aim to reduce altitude illness with a careful acclimatisation schedule, reserving medication for emergency treatment where possible. While competitive climbing is a regulated sport, recreational trekking and mountaineering are not.

Further reading

Johnson, C., Anderson, S.R., Dallimore, J. *et al.* (2014) *Oxford Handbook of Expedition and Wilderness Medicine*, 2nd edn. Oxford University Press, Oxford. *A fantastic pocket sized 'Oxford Handbook' covering the spectrum of medicine in austere environments – also available as an iPhone/iPad app.*

Luks, A.M., McIntosh, S.E., Grissom, C.K. *et al.* (2010) Wilderness medical society consensus guidelines for the prevention and treatment of acute altitude illness. *Wilderness & Environmental Medicine*, **21**, 146–155.

Medex. *Travel at High Altitude*. 2nd ed. Medex, 2008. Available from www.medex.org.uk. *Easy to read and suitable for both medical personnel and trekkers/athletes. Free downloads available in a variety of languages & an iPad version. Recommended for anyone contemplating any activity at high altitude.*

Pedlar C, Whyte G, Kreindler K, Hardman S and Levine, B. The BASES expert statement on human performance in hypoxia inducing environments: natural and simulated altitude. Concise review of altitude training strategies available from http://www.bases.org.uk/BASES-Expert-Statements. Accessed 19 June 2015.

Pollard, A.J. & Murdoch, D.R. (2003) *The High Altitude Medicine Handbook*, 3rd edn. Radcliffe Medical Press, Abingdon. *Hard to obtain, but an excellent resource designed for both medical and lay readers.*

UIAA – International Climbing and Mountaineering Federation Medical Commission Advice & Recommendations. Available from http://www.theuiaa.org/medical_advice.html. *Fantastic free evidence based advice in a variety of languages.* Accessed 19 June 2015.

Wagner, D.R. (2012) Medical and sporting ethics of high altitude mountaineering: the use of drugs and supplemental oxygen. *Wilderness & Environmental Medicine*, **23**, 205–206.

West, J.B., Schoene, R.B., Luks, A.M. & Milledge, J.S. (2012) *High Altitude Medicine and Physiology*, 5th edn. CRC Press, Boca Raton. *The definitive textbook – a tremendous resource for the dedicated high altitude physician or researcher, but probably too in-depth for most.*

World Anti-doping Agency. Available from http://www.wada-ama.org/en/. *Sports medicine physicians should be familiar with both the Code and the latest Prohibited List.* Accessed 19 June 2015.

CHAPTER 17

Physical Activity and Exercise as Medicine

John Buckley

Institute of Medicine, University Centre Shrewsbury and University of Chester, Chester, UK

OVERVIEW

In this chapter we describe the role of physical activity in medicine. After studying this chapter, the reader will know

- The fundamentals to increasing physical activity
- Changing sedentary behaviours
- Risk reduction and physical activity
- Exercise prescription
- Exercise intensity and health outcomes

Hippocrates in the 4th century BC put forth the concept of both natural and artificial exercises as a means for better health. The former occurring in daily life (for transport, occupation and domestic living) and the latter is performed in one's leisure time (sport, exercise, recreational pursuits). In the 1950s and 1960s, studies by Morris and Paffenbarger were the first to scientifically demonstrate a link between health, disease and occupational levels of physical (in) activity. There is now an immerging evidence base showing that it is not just increased activity that has a preventive effect for health. Spending long periods of time sitting, independent of one's levels of exercise, is now a significant risk factor for cardiometabolic disease, some cancers and mental health.

A key historical example of exercise as secondary preventive medicine was reported by Dr William Heberden FRCP (the man who defined angina pectoris), when in 1772 he noted a cure for angina was exercise when a patient sawed wood for 30 min per day. The biological mechanisms to why exercise improves arterial/endothelial function and integrity have only become more fully understood since the year 2000.

It is interesting and important to note that in all of the above original historical examples of physical activity linked to health or disease, the mode of activity was occupational and not leisure time exercise or sport. This demonstrates the importance or influence that activities inherent within daily life are a significant component to health and not to be overlooked even when people participate in regular exercise training. Globally, reducing physical inactivity has become one of nine key health targets of the World Health Organisation (WHO). A special edition of the *Lancet* prepared for WHO prior to the 2012 London Olympics Games highlighted that globally physical inactivity is prevalent in 40% of those with cardiovascular disease, diabetes and some cancers. Alarmingly, this prevalence rises to 70% in western European countries, including the United Kingdom. Less sitting, caused by the modern built and social environments, is therefore as important to health as increased physical activity, exercise and sports participation.

The ABC of *Gearing-up* behaviour for increasing physical activity

The *ABC* elements to physical activity behaviour include the following:

A. Simply avoiding too much sitting
B. Increasing opportunities to walk and move more in daily life
C. Focused exercise training, sports participation and active leisure pursuits

The rationale for points A and B is that over the past five decades, there has been a loss of ~200 kcals per day of energy expenditure in people's lives at work, at home, during leisure time and as part of transport. Standing compared to sitting has a differential energy expenditure between 0.5 and 1.0 kcal min^{-1}, and simply standing a total of two extra hours per day would equate to 25,000 kcals per year. Focused exercise training (point C) provides the strongest health and clinical outcomes in both primary and secondary preventions for all key chronic conditions, but for most people (>70% of the population) it continues to be too great a behavioural challenge.

Figure 17.1 illustrates the continuum of activity from a sedentary state to more vigorous intensity exercise training, with the percentages of how much of the British public's waking hours are spent at each level. The British population spends 60–70% of their waking hours sitting, noted as being in 'reverse' gear (R). Simply standing and moving about or easy walking are considered light activity (first and second gear), which now makes up most of the developed world's physical activity; however, only 20–30% of people's waking hours are spent in this mode. Moderate intensity activity (third gear), which physiologically demands at least 40–50%

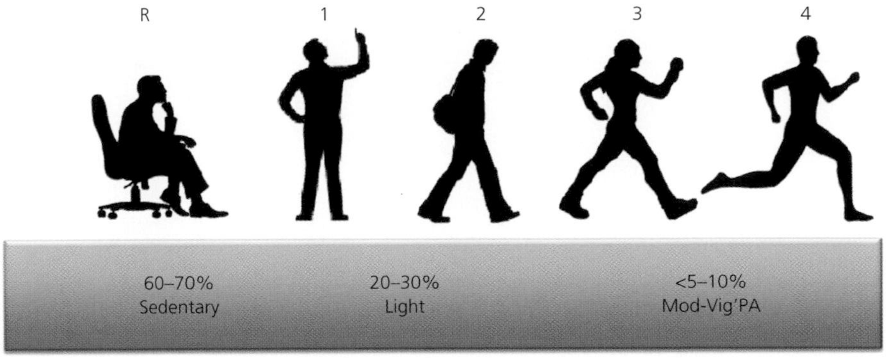

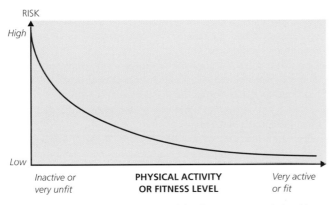

Figure 17.1 Proportion of weekly waking hours spent in activity modes, ranging from time spent sitting through to vigorous physical activity (Adapted from Townsend *et al.*,). Values *R*, 1, 2, 3 and 4 represent behavioural 'gears' synonymous to a car, where *R* = 'reverse', 1 and 2 = light activities within daily living, 3 and 4 are moderate to vigorous activities either in daily life or as part of leisure-time pursuits, exercise and sport

Figure 17.2 Schematic representation of the dose–response relationship between physical activity level and risk of disease. This curvilinear dose–response curve generally holds for coronary heart disease and type 2 diabetes: the higher the level of physical activity or fitness, the lower the risk of disease. Curves for other diseases will become more apparent as the volume of evidence increases. Source: Department of Health, Chief Medical Officers 2011. Crown Copyright

of maximum aerobic capacity (VO_{2max}), is the minimum level required to achieve improved cardio-respiratory fitness. Vigorous to high-intensity training (fourth gear) demonstrates the greatest physiological benefit in improving fitness when performed three or more times per week. However, moderate to vigorous activity currently makes up less than 10% of people's weekly waking hours (5–20 min per day).

Figure 17.2 illustrates that the greatest relative risk reduction for highly sedentary people occurs in moving to simply being on their feet more and performing more walking. The model in Figure 17.1 illustrates this as moving from reverse gear into first and second gears. In those who claim to 'being on their feet most of the day', they should then be encouraged and supported to partake in more moderate to vigorous activity (third and fourth gear). All too often people who have a desire to become more active by taking up moderate to vigorous exercise pursuits fail to maintain such a change and the behaviour literally stalls; synonymous to taking a car from reverse gear straight into third or fourth gear, the engine will stall. In those who are successful in maintaining regular moderate to vigorous activity of 150 min per week, they must still avoid sitting too much the rest of the day as it has now been shown to cancel out much of the risk reduction benefit of the exercise.

Exercise training

Much of the focus thus far has highlighted the ills of sedentary behaviour and potential benefits of moving large swathes of the population into frequent bouts of light activity. However, in those able to meet the more ideal behaviour of regular moderate to vigorous exercise, they should be guided by the best available evidence. Over the past three decades, most of the guidance has been on continuous aerobic exercise performed 3–5 days per week, at an intensity between 40 and 75% of aerobic capacity (VO_{2max}), for 20–60 min. Within such guidance, a more precise and individualised means of setting intensity would be to set target work rates or heart rates at the ventilatory, anaerobic or lactate threshold. Table 17.1 provides a summary of more practical means of setting exercise intensity using heart rate and ratings of perceived exertion. Additionally, national physical activity guidelines now include strength training being performed 2 or more days per week, with intensities in the region of 50–70% 1-repetition maximum (1RM), for 10–15 repetitions over 1–3 sets, and applied to 8–10 muscle groups.

Continuous and interval-type training

Emerging evidence for greater health and fitness gains is increasingly being reported for those employing lower volume high-intensity interval training (HIIT). Historically, however, this approach has been used since the 1930s for athletic training. Benefits, safety and efficacy have even been shown in some studies involving patients with established cardiovascular disease. Although the science of these studies on HIIT are quite compelling in terms of efficacy and safety in widening participation to larger populations, there are a number of pragmatic, physical, psychological and social challenges that need to be considered, including

- Participants in studies did not have other limiting co-morbidities, which are typically present in older or clinical populations.
- All individuals received specialised screening, maximal testing and close supervision during the trials.
- Trials were short term; would individuals wish to continue and enjoy performing this style of training in the long-term?
- Exercise and physical activity are social pursuits, for which people may be concerned less about shortening sessions because of enjoying their time with others.
- Long-term health outcomes are yet to be reported.

Table 17.1 Practical means of expressing relative intensities for aerobic exercise

%VO$_{2max}$[a] % HR reserve[b,c]	%HR$_{max}$[c,d]	Perceived exertion descriptor[d]	Borg RPE (6–20 Scale)[d]	Borg RPE (CR10 scale)[e]
28	50	Very light	9	1
42	60	Light	11	2
56	70	Somewhat hard	12–13	3.0–3.5
70	80	Somewhat hard	13–14	3.5–4.5
83	90	Hard	15–16	5.5–6.5
100	100	Maximal	19	10

[a]Percentage of maximal aerobic power (%VO$_{2max}$) can generally be represented by the same percentage of heart rate reserve (%HR reserve). Lactate or ventilatory thresholds typically occur at 40–55% VO$_{2max}$ in inactive or newly commencing participants; 56–75% for regularly and moderately trained individuals, and >75% VO$_{2max}$ for more highly trained individuals.
[b]The Karvonen method is used to determine heart rate reserve where both resting heart rate and maximal heart rate are required in the calculation, which aims to accommodate for differences in resting heart rates, especially for older or clinical populations.
[c]Ideally maximal heart rate should be determined from a maximal exercise test, but can be estimated by the following:

   a. In healthy individuals using Tanaka *et al.* equation: 208–0.7 × age
   b. In older or clinical populations Inbar *et al.* equation: 206–0.7 × age
   c. Subtract 20–30 beats per minute for those on beta-blockade or on Ivabradine
   d. In beta-blocked heart failure patients, with chronotropic incompetence using the Keteyian equation: 119 + 0.5 (resting HR) − 0.5 (age), with further −5 beats per minute if exercise is on a cycle ergometer.

[d]Descriptors and values on Borg's 6–20 rating of perceived exertion (RPE) scale.
[e]Borg's category ratio (CR10) scale, which is more sensitive for those with specific symptoms, for example, breathlessness, vascular disease pain, muscle pain.
Source: Data from BACPR manual and ACPICR Standards

In health and clinical populations most of the trials have focused on the benefits of exercise for single conditions, with significant effects. However, in reality many individuals live with multiple risk factors and the available evidence for the collective benefits of HIIT exercise across a group of risk factors that an individual may requires further evaluation. Long-term adherence to exercise have strongly correlated with mood, sense of enjoyment and self-efficacy, where exercise practitioners must balance the consideration of these elements equally with the scientific physiological parameters.

Summary

Overall health gains from being physically active are likely to come from a number of strategies, which are adapted to individual circumstances of domestic life, occupation, time, beliefs and motivation. The built and social environment, historically, have been the key factors affecting sedentary behaviour. More effort is needed to help influence people becoming more active from a starting point of simply sitting less within daily life, in parallel with finding acceptable means of regular participation in moderate to vigorous intensity activities.

Further reading

ACPICR. *Standards for Physical Activity and Exercise in the Cardiac Population* London: Association of Chartered Physiotherapists in Cardiac Rehabilitation, 2015 www.acpicr.com.

BACPR (2014) *A Practical Approach to Exercise and Physical Activity in the Prevention and Management of Cardiovascular Disease*. British Association for Cardiovascular Prevention and Rehabilitation, London.

Biddle, S.J. & Mutrie, N. (2008) *Psychology of Physical Activity*, 2nd edn. Routledge, London and New York.

Buckley, J.P., Mellor, D.D., Morris, M. & Joseph, F. (2014) Standing-based office work shows encouraging signs of attenuating post-prandial glycaemic excursion. *Occupational and Environmental Medicine*, **71**, 109–111.

Church, T.S., Thomas, D.M., Tudor-Locke, C. *et al.* (2011) Trends over 5 decades in U.S. occupation-related physical activity and their associations with obesity. *PLoS One*, **6**, e19657.

Dempsey, P.C., Owen, N., Biddle, S.J. & Dunstan, D.W. (2014) Managing sedentary behavior to reduce the risk of diabetes and cardiovascular disease. *Current Diabetes Reports*, **14**, 522.

Department of Health, Chief Medical Officers. Start Active Stay Active; a report on physical activity from the four home countries' Chief Medical Officers. 2011.

Maher, C., Olds, T., Mire, E. & Katzmarzyk, P.T. (2014) Reconsidering the sedentary behaviour paradigm. *PLoS One*, **9**, e86403.

Mann, T., Lamberts, R.P. & Lambert, M.I. (2013) Methods of prescribing relative exercise intensity: physiological and practical considerations. *Sports Medicine*, **43**, 613–625.

W.H.O. Prevention and control of noncommunicable diseases: formal meeting of Member States to conclude the work on the comprehensive global monitoring framework, including indicators, and a set of voluntary global targets for the prevention and control of noncommunicable diseases; Report by the Director-General of the World Health Organisation. 2012, p. 3–9.

CHAPTER 18

Sport, Exercise and Disability

Nick Webborn

Centre for Sport and Exercise Science and Medicine (SESAME), University of Brighton, Eastbourne, East Sussex, UK

OVERVIEW

In this chapter we describe the area of sport, exercise and disability. After studying this chapter, the reader will know

- Participation and Paralympic sport
- Eligibility and classification
- Selecting disability sport
- Injury risk
- Anti-doping considerations

Box 18.1 **Changes in sport participation/interest**

- Local Government Association survey in March 2013 showed 5% of councils saw a large increase in leisure/gym users with a disability, and 28% a small increase.
- Eight out of 10 disabled people are considering taking up sport following the Games (C4 and English Federation for Disability Sport).
- Seventy percentage of disabled people agree that the London 2012 Paralympic Games was inspirational for them (C4 and English Federation of Disability Sport (EFDS)).

The Chief Medical Officers report on Physical Activity for Health outlines recommendations on safe physical activity and also acknowledges that barriers related to gender, ethnicity, disability and access still need to be addressed. There is accumulating evidence that people with disabilities who are more physically active tend to have fewer visits to physicians, have fewer complications and hospitalisations than their sedentary counterparts and so the promotion of physical activity health is essential. The principles of training, for example, the graded increase in duration, intensity and frequency of activity, apply the same to people with disabilities but more thought may be required as to the mode of exercise according to the impairment and potential complicating factors. The social and psychological benefits of exercise and sport participation are not exclusive to the able-bodied, and major improvements in self-esteem and social integration may occur through an active lifestyle in disabled people. Also the lessons and experiences from elite Paralympic sport can shed light on the modes of activity suitable for people with a disability and also provide cautions in relation to emerging data on injury in relation to participation.

Increasing participation and resources

While barriers do remain to participation in sport and physical activity, there have been some significant steps forward. The British Paralympic Association developed a website (www.parasport.org .uk) to facilitate finding an appropriate sport for a particular

---

Box 18.2 **Educational toolkit topics**

- Fit for life – exercise and health information
- How to overcome barriers to exercise
- Physical activity and exercise-specific guides and cautions
- Nutrition

---

impairment type or to locate a local club by postcode search. Following the 2012 Paralympic Games, there has been a 400% increase in hits from people trying to find a club local to them. There was greater than 700% increase in people using the self-assessment tool on the website to find a suitable sport for their particular impairment type. Additionally, during the period of games, 800 new clubs loaded their information onto the parasport website (Box 18.1).

However, sporting activity is not necessary and not necessarily the preferred way of getting physical activity for many people. The Peter Harrison Centre for Disability Sport has developed a series of educational toolkits (Box 18.2; www.lboro.ac.uk/research/phc/). These provide disability-specific guides to help people understand how to lead a healthy, active lifestyle. The educational toolkits have been developed for people with the Paralympic medical impairment groups (see Table 18.1) with disability-specific advice.

Paralympic sports

The success of the London 2012 Paralympic Games thrust the achievements of people with a disability into the spotlight with

---

ABC of Sports and Exercise Medicine, Fourth Edition.
Edited by Gregory P. Whyte, Mike Loosemore and Clyde Williams.
© 2015 John Wiley & Sons, Ltd. Published 2015 by John Wiley & Sons, Ltd.

Table 18.1 List of paralympic summer sports, impairment group, international federation and dates

Sport	Impairment categories	Governing body	Paralympic Games status
Archery	AMP, LA, CP, SCRD	FITA	(1960–present)
Athletics	AMP, LA, CP, ID, VI, SCRD	IPC	(1960–present)
Boccia	CP	CP-ISRA	(1984–present)
Canoe	AMP, LA, CP, SCRD	ICF	Starting 2016
Cycling	AMP, LA, CP, VI, SCRD	UCI	(1988–present)
Equestrian	AMP, LA, CP, VI, SCRD	FEI	(1996–present)
Football 5-a-Side	VI	IBSA	(2004–present)
Football 7-a-Side	CP	CP-ISRA	(1984–present)
Goalball	VI	IBSA	(1980–present)
Judo	VI	IBSA	(1988–present)
Powerlifting	AMP, LA, CP, SCRD	IPC	(1964–present)
Rowing	AMP, LA, CP, VI, SCRD	FISA	(2008–present)
Sailing	AMP, LA, CP, VI, SCRD	IFDS	(2000–present)
Shooting	AMP, LA, CP, VI, SCRD	IPC	(1976–present)
Swimming	AMP, LA, CP, ID, VI, SCRD	IPC	(1960–present)
Table tennis	AMP, LA, CP, SCRD	ITTF	(1960–present)
Triathlon	AMP, LA, CP, VI, SCRD	ITU	Starting 2016
Volleyball	AMP, LA	WOVD	(1976–present)
Wheelchair basketball	SCRD, AMP, LA	IWBF	(1960–present)
Wheelchair fencing	SCRD	IWAS	(1960–present)
Wheelchair rugby	SCRD	IWRF	(2000–present)
Wheelchair tennis	SCRD	ITF	(1992–present)

Key: Spinal cord-related disability – SCRD, VI – visually impaired, AMP – amputee, CP – cerebral palsy, LA – Les Autres, LD – learning difficulties.

unprecedented media coverage. This led to not only a change in perception of the public with regard to people with disability but also evidence of increasing participation in physical activity and sport by people with disabilities as a consequence. Competitive sport for people with a disability involved from an archery contest for people with spinal cord injury on the lawns of Stoke Mandeville Hospital in 1948 to become the second largest sporting event in the world with over 4000 participants from 164 participating nations, competing in 20 different sports and viewed by over 2.7 million paying spectators. There will be 22 summer sports in the 2016 Games with para-canoe and para-triathlon as new sports (see Table 18.1). There are also five winter Paralympic sports. Paralympic sports developed either as adaptations of an able-bodied equivalent sport, or as one devised to accommodate the impairment type with no able-bodied equivalent.

Eligibility and classification

To participate in a Paralympic sport, one must have an eligible impairment of sufficient severity for inclusion. Then athletes are classified into different levels of impairment for fairer competition. As Paralympic sport evolved, it moved away from a traditional medical model of classification by medical impairment type to a more detailed study of the impact of the impairment on the ability to perform the sport. The major medical issues by impairment type are shown in Box 18.3, while the list of eligible impairment types is shown is Box 18.4. However, the medical diagnosis remains important from the perspective of planning healthcare for events or athlete team care by understanding fully the potential medical complications and injury patterns.

Box 18.3 **Medical impairment types**

- Amputation/limb deficiency
- Cerebral palsy (CP)
- Spinal-cord-related disability (SCRD)
- 'Les Autres (LA)' – used to describe physical impairments not fitting in above types
- Visual impairment
- Intellectual impairment

Box 18.4 **Eligible impairment types**

- Hypertonia
- Ataxia
- Athetosis
- Loss of muscle strength
- Loss of range of movement
- Loss of limb
- Limb deficiency
- Short stature
- Low vision
- Intellectual impairment

Source: Data from International Paralympic Committee (IPC) Classification Code 2007

Choosing a sport or activity

People with disabilities can take part in virtually every sport available including high-risk sports such as mountain climbing, sub-aqua diving and skiing. Some sports are conventional sports in which little or no modification is required, for example, swimming. Other sports may require specific adaptation, for example, wheelchair basketball, or may be specifically developed for a certain disability, for example, goalball for the visually impaired (VI). In helping to choose a sport or activity, it is important to establish the individual's aims. If the aim is primarily for physical health benefits for a general health or disease modification, then one has to consider the difference between exercise and sport. These terms are often incorrectly used interchangeably. Sport is not always exercise and vice versa. Sport implies competition, and the physiological demands are determined by the sport, for example, wheelchair sprint racing (anaerobic) vs wheelchair road racing (aerobic) vs pistol shooting (skill). Sport may also involve trauma, which will be particularly undesirable in some medical conditions. Alternatively, the focus may be on socialisation and building self-esteem. While the ability to achieve one of these aims is not necessarily exclusive of the others, it is helpful to consider the person's goals and the risk of participation. Not all sports need to be organised or competitive. The choice of sport will be influenced by various factors (Box 18.5).

Injury risk

All sporting participation carries the potential for injury. The risk is individual to each sport and Paralympic sports are no different. There is however the potential for injury in a Paralympic athlete to have a greater impact on the ability to perform activities of daily living and longer term consequences to health. For example, the wheelchair athlete who injures their shoulder may have difficulty in performing basic transfers to and from their wheelchair affecting quality of life. The largest cohort study of injury in Paralympic sport captured data of nearly 50,000 athlete days of exposure. The results showed an overall injury rate of 12.7 injuries/1000 athlete days but with wide variation between sports with the highest injury rates seen in Football 5-a-side, goalball and powerlifting. Injuries in the upper limb predominated, but there are clear sport-specific determinants of injury risk and area of injury, for example, lower limb injuries associated with collision with an opponent was the predominant cause of acute competition injury in Football 5-a-side.

The specificity by sport information is crucial when considering prevention strategies.

Anti-doping considerations

The IPC is a signatory of the World Anti-Doping Code and the principle of 'strict liability' applies equally in Paralympic sport. Historically, doping has not been a major problem in Paralympic sport. Unfortunately, the sport of powerlifting does have a history of adverse analytical results for prohibited substances, particularly with anabolic agents where strength gains from their use can improve performance. The Therapeutic Use Exemption process must be followed for athletes with disabilities who may have co-existing conditions that require the use of, for example, strong analgesics or diuretics.

Sample collection is an area of difference in Paralympic athletes. The use of catheters for collection of the sample is permitted, but urine may not be collected from a leg bag without prior emptying in the doping control station as substitution of urine could have occurred. Athletes with a visual or intellectual impairment require supervision by an accompanying person to ensure integrity of the sample.

Medical education and training

Historically, relatively few practitioners had experience in the medical aspects of sport for people with disabilities. However, the awarding of the 2012 Olympic and Paralympic Games to London saw the creation of the speciality of Sport and Exercise Medicine in the United Kingdom. The curriculum for specialty training in Sport and Exercise Medicine includes a specific module on 'Spinal Injuries, Amputee Rehabilitation & Disability Sport', which is also a component in the Diploma of Sport and Exercise Medicine Examination (UK). Consequently, we have a generation of emerging specialists and diplomats with knowledge, skills and experience in the discipline. Approximately 100 doctors gained experience in the area as volunteers at the Paralympic Games in London. This growing group of practitioners through experience in athlete care will now be better prepared to help advise on and promote physical activity for non-athletes with disabilities as well (Figure 18.1).

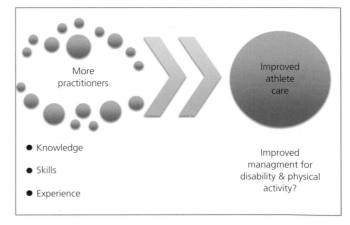

Figure 18.1 List of summer Paralympic sports by impairment group, international federation and date

Summary

Paralympic sport has moved on significantly in terms of levels of performance and recognition and perception by the public (Box 18.6). There are also more suitable facilities available and a variety of resources to aid people to find local clubs and other educational resources.

These experiences now need to lead to a more general improvement in promotion of physical activity for people with disabilities.

Further reading

Thompson, W.R. & Vanlandewijck, Y. (2011) *The Paralympic Athlete*. Wiley Blackwell, Oxford.

Van De Vliet, P. (2011) Event medical care for paralympic athletes. In: McDonagh, D., O'Sullivan, L.J., Frontera, W.R., Pigozzi, F., Grimm, K., Butler, C.F., *et al.* (eds), *FIMS Sports Medicine Manual Event Planning and Emergency Care*. Lippincott Williams & Wilkins, Philadelphia.

Webborn, A.D.J. (2009) Paralympic sports. In: Caine, D.J., Harmer, P.A. & Schiff, M.A. (eds), *Epidemiology of Injury in Olympic Sports*. Wiley-Blackwell, Oxford, UK, pp. 437–488.

CHAPTER 19

Sport, Exercise and Obesity

David Haslam

National Obesity Forum, Luton and Dunstable NHS Trust, Dunstable Road, Luton, UK

OVERVIEW

In this chapter we describe the role of sport and exercise in obesity. After studying this chapter, the reader will know

- Physical activity guidelines
- The impact of physical activity on obesity and mortality
- Childhood and geriatric obesity and exercise
- Physical activity versus diet in the control of obesity
- The role of exercise and obesity

Introduction

Obesity is associated with the co-existence of serious non-communicable disease and premature mortality. Physical activity is widely associated with the opposite: a broad spectrum of health gains across many areas of well-being. Our prehistoric ancestors were equipped to conserve energy as a precious commodity; physical activity was needed to hunt for food and to avoid becoming something else's food. Resting between onerous bouts of exercise was important for the survival of the species. Modern man has inherited the tendency to sedentariness, and the obesogenic environment has all but obliterated the need to be active, causing an imbalance in energy expenditure compared to energy consumption which is now one of the many causes of the current obesity epidemic. The decline in physical activity is strongly linked to the significant fall in free-living and vocational activities. The extra physical activity involved in daily living 50 years ago compared with today has been estimated to be the equivalent of running a marathon per week. Furthermore, only 20% of men and 10% of women have physically active occupations.

Physical activity guidelines

Most guidelines, such as those of the World Health Organisation (WHO), are based on public health principles of maintaining good health, given that two-thirds of the population already suffers from excess weight is of limited value. Current guidelines suggest that to stay healthy, adults aged 19–64 years should try to be active daily and should do at least 150 min of moderate intensity aerobic activity such as cycling or fast walking every week, and muscle-strengthening activities on 2 or more days a week that work all major muscle groups (legs, hips, back, abdomen, chest, shoulders and arms). Alternatively, guidelines suggest that 75 min of vigorous intensity aerobic activity can be used to substitute for moderate intensity activity.

Of note, short, frequent periods of exercise attenuate glucose excursions and insulin concentrations in obese individuals to a greater degree than an equal amount of exercise performed continuously in the morning. Furthermore, one bout of physical activity reduces average glucose and post-prandial glucose within hours. This has led to the suggestion that shorter episodes of a minimum of 10 min performed frequently across the day are effective in promoting health.

The WHO report on Diet, Nutrition and Prevention of Chronic Diseases concluded that between 60 and 90 min of moderate intensity physical activity per day is required to lose weight or prevent weight regain after substantial loss. Individuals with sedentary occupations should ensure that periods of sitting are broken at least every 30 min by some form of activity. The optimum degree of exertion is said to be that which raises the pulse, causes sweating and quickened breathing, but with the person still able to talk. This is often termed 'brisk' exercise. However, this must be in addition to routine activities of daily living, that is, light-intensity tasks, such as self-care, walking, shopping or gardening.

At least 10,000 steps per day (as monitored on a pedometer) are recommended for maintenance of health. 15,000 steps are required to lose weight or maintain weight loss, although for many this is impractical, and for others impossible. It is important to note that for an obese, inactive individual, an initial increase from 0 to 200 steps a day will have substantial health benefits. For disabled individuals, that is, anyone who cannot walk 10,000 steps because of any disability, the US Surgeon General's report recommends wheeling in a wheelchair for 40 min as being a reasonable level of activity for health benefits. Additional exercise alone, nutritional changes, will more often than not imp without any accompanying weight loss due to t of fat to muscle. Total fat has been show

ABC of Sports and Exercise Medicine, Fourth Edition.
Edited by Gregory P. Whyte, Mike Loosemore and Clyde Williams.

different in fat-fit and fat-unfit individuals, but visceral fat and liver fat are significantly lower in the fat-fit than the fat-unfit.

Most adults are insufficiently active; 75% of adults get less activity than advised. Fifty-six percentage of men believe that they are sufficiently active to benefit their health, whereas in fact only 36% approach even moderate activity. Similarly, 52% of women believe they do enough exercise, but only 24% reach recommended guidelines for physical activity. A sedentary individual will burn off 25% of daily energy expenditure on physical activity, the rest going on thermogenesis and basal metabolism. In contrast, elite athletes will use up to 80% of energy expenditure on physical activity. It has been demonstrated that an obese child sitting motionless in front of the television can be so inert that he burns off energy at less than basal metabolic rate (BMR). Different ethnic groups follow physical activity recommendations to different extents: only 37% of black Caribbean men, 30% of Indian men and 26% of Bangladeshi men are 'sufficiently' active, compared with 37% of the general male population. In women, 11% of Bangladeshi women, 23% of Indian women and 31% of black Caribbean women meet the recommendations, compared with 25% of the general population.

Physical activity, obesity and mortality

Beneficial effects of activity on mortality have been demonstrated in a large number of studies from around the globe. The National Institutes of Health, American Association of Retired Persons Diet and Health Study, which included 252,925 subjects, reported that those individuals adhering to the national physical activity guidelines exhibited lower risk of death than others who were inactive. Individuals who met recommendations for moderate activity decreased their mortality risk by 27%, whereas in those who met recommendations for vigorous activity demonstrated a 32% reduction.

Another prospective study performed two fitness assessments in each of almost 10,000 men at a mean interval of 4.9 years and evaluated the effect of change, or lack of change, in physical fitness on mortality. The highest all-cause and cardiovascular mortality rate was in men who were unfit at both examinations, whereas men who were fit on both occasions exhibited lowest mortality. Men who improved from unfit to fit, benefitted from a reduction in all-cause mortality risk of 44% and of cardiovascular mortality by 52% compared to those who remained unfit at both examinations. In elderly adults followed up for 6 years, free-living activity is strongly associated with a reduced risk of all-cause mortality. Free-living activity expending ~287 kcal per day reduces risk of mortality by 30%.

Childhood obesity and exercise

Twenty-first century existence has affected children just as much as adults; the morning walk to school is a rarity, as parents become increasingly concerned about pollution and child safety. A 2013 study showed that only 25% of primary school children in England are allowed to travel home from school alone compared with 86% in 1971. Physical activity at school has reduced as successive governments have sold off playing fields, condemned competitive

sports as socially and politically unacceptable, and bowed to an increasingly litigious society by not putting children at the slightest risk of injury. Home is safer and more comfortable than ever; on average children watch 3 h of television per day. The risk of becoming overweight is 4.6 times higher in children who watch more than 5 h of television per day. Reducing sedentary time such as watching TV is more beneficial in weight management than attempting to introduce vigorous activity sessions. In the United States Children, it has been demonstrated that obesity relates directly to the number of hour spent watching television with 3 h per day doubling the risk of obesity and type 2 diabetes. In the United Kingdom, almost 50% of girls and 38% of boys do not achieve a single 10-min period of activity equivalent to brisk walking across three school days. The importance of this epidemic of inactivity in childhood was highlighted in a recent study that permitted students to stay in bed resting for 60 days. Their visceral adipose stores increased by 29%, fat tissue in the remainder of the trunk, from chin to the iliac crest by10%, and in the arms and legs by 7% alongside a reduction in insulin sensitivity.

Geriatric obesity and exercise

Physical activity levels, not surprisingly, decline with age; elderly patients often suffer from low muscle mass with surplus ectopic fat within their muscle (sarcopenia) and viscera. An elderly individual with any given BMI will usually have a higher percentage of body fat mass than a younger counterpart with similar BMI. Accordingly, increased physical activity of any degree should be promoted in an ageing population. A recent meta-analysis commented that many frail older adults are thin, weak and undernourished, but there is also strong evidence that excessive adiposity contributes to frailty by reducing the ability of older adults to perform physical activities and increasing metabolic instability.

Physical activity versus diet in the control of obesity

The EarlyBird study of childhood obesity reports interesting and counter-intuitive observations. It is a large prospective cohort study of healthy children from the age of 5 years. The study found that the average pre-pubertal child is no heavier now than when children were assessed for the 1990 UK growth standard charts: mean BMI has risen, but the median very little, suggesting that a sub-group of children skews the distribution without altering its position. Data suggest that the rise in childhood obesity involves the sons of obese fathers, who have a sixfold greater risk, and daughters of obese mothers, who have a 10-fold greater risk; but not vice versa. EarlyBird describes an 'activitystat' which operates to defend a child's activity set-point. In-school Physical Activity-intense children record 40% more activity during school hours, but recorded correspondingly less outside of school on arriving home, such that the totals over the course of the whole day were the same in all groups, irrespective of opportunity. This compensatory response suggests that physical activity of children may be controlled by the brain, rather than the environment, and that children compensate accordingly. The study introduced the concept of children being movers or non-movers, who will compensate adequately for either enforced sedentariness or enforced activity by doing the precise opposite during the remainder of the day. Most importantly, physical inactivity does not lead to obesity, but instead, obesity to inactivity, suggesting again that the primary cause of childhood obesity is overnutrition and implying that weight loss might of itself lead to more activity and better metabolic health.

Residential activity programmes, once known as 'Fat Camps', are usually for obese children and adolescents, and involve intensive supervised activity. Detractors have argued that camps are only brief excursions away from a person's usual environment, any reduction in body weight will be transient and reverse when the person returns to the normal daily routine. They comment that the cohort of attenders are self-selecting, representing the minority of children who have both motivation and funding to attend.

However, others argue that weight-loss diets are potentially unsafe in children and so increased activity is essential, and that management strategies that combine dietary education, behavioural modification, a reduction in sedentary pursuits and an increase in physical activity are likely to succeed. The emphasis in camps is on enjoyment of activity, so that there is a chance for it to continue at home. There are three elements:

- Fun-type exercise and physical activities
- Skill development in the physical activities
- Exposure of children to a wide range of physical activities with a strong element of choice

Studies demonstrate favourable changes in body mass, adiposity and other risk factors following attendance allowing optimistic predictions for the future of residential activity programmes.

Appetite, exercise and obesity

Appetite control, to an extent, may be governed by long-term fitness; 'fit' individuals who exercise regularly have 'normal' appetites, whereas sedentary 'unfit' people lose regulatory control due to the lack of the normal stimuli and exercise pattern ingrained during our hunting, gathering past. The exact reasons are not known; however, it has been suggested that active people rely on hunger to tell them when to eat and therefore control food intake, whereas inactive individuals rely on satiety to tell them when they are replenished: hunger is a more efficient physiological mechanism than satiety; therefore active individuals control weight better.

Exercise and obesity

The additional amount of weight lost by diet and physical activity, compared with diet alone, can be relatively low, but the medical benefits of physical activity are highly significant, because regular exercise induces increase in muscle bulk at the expense of fat, which results in an increased fat-free mass: muscle weighs one-and-a-half times as much as fat, so actual body weight may be maintained or may even increase when patients initiate exercise regimes. Increasing muscle tissue increases BMR, in contrast to the reduction in BMR that usually occurs with weight loss, thus assisting simultaneous dietary efforts to lose weight.

It has long been known that physical activity has significant health benefits over and above weight loss (Table 19.1).

A landmark study in the early 1990s examined contrasting patterns of energy expenditure over 1 day for a sedentary person, a person who engage in scheduled vigorous exercise during a lunchtime break, but was otherwise sedentary, and an individual with a sedentary job with short bouts of routine daily physical activity throughout the day. The energy expenditure was greatest for the latter individual and should prompt clinicians to favour the approach of promoting routine activity across the day as successful and sustainable.

While traditional forms of exercise may be acceptable for some obese individuals, physical activities as part of daily living are often a better, more acceptable concept, that is, daily chores such as gardening and cleaning can meaningfully contribute to an overall daily calorie output. So it is important that activity is not exclusively linked to scheduled exercise sessions such as gym sessions or sporting fixtures: although these are excellent ways to obtain exercise, and commercial gyms may be a suitable way of losing weight and improving fitness for some. Despite the significant increase in the private gym sector with 8 million members in the United Kingdom, obesity levels have risen. There are a range of reasons underpinning this lack of impact including the high number (over 50% in the United States) of health club members residing in the top 20% of income earners, whereas deprived groups, excluded from this market, were most likely to be inactive and therefore obese.

Thus, exercise and activity should be promoted on an individual basis. It is important to advise individuals to begin gently and increase slowly, and to ensure they will continue with activity, they should be encouraged to choose an enjoyable form compatible with their physical condition, so they are more likely to continue and gain benefit. All health professionals including pharmacists, midwives, and nurses, can play a key role in advising parents and children to take part in activity so that it may become a life-long habit.

For weight loss, the optimal exercise is often considered to be moderate intensity, using oxidation of free fatty acids for energy. Activities such as swimming, brisk walking, gardening, wheeling in a wheelchair to burn off fat, combined with a reduced calorie intake, are most effective for weight reduction and for maintenance of weight loss (see Tables 19.2 and 19.3). The more prolonged the activity, the more oxidation of fat occurs for use as an energy source, and there is evidence that fat stores are oxidised after prolonged bouts of exercise to top up reduced glycogen stores.

Table 19.1 Health benefits of physical activity in obese individuals

- Improved control of type 2 diabetes
- Improvement in lipid profile, in particular increase in high density lipoproteins (HDL)
- Improved control of blood pressure
- Enhanced insulin sensitivity
- Better self-esteem and attenuated symptoms of depression
- Improved day-to-day functional capacity
- Reduced risk of colorectal cancer due to altered metabolism of environmental carcinogens

Table 19.2 Examples of moderate intensity physical activity

- Brisk walking
- Cycling
- Swimming (with moderate effort)
- Stair climbing (with moderate effort)
- Gardening: digging, pushing mower or sweeping leaves
- General house cleaning
- Painting and decorating
- General callisthenics (sit-ups, push-ups, chin-ups)
- Gentle racquet sports such as table tennis and badminton (social)
- Golf walking, wheeling or carrying clubs

Table 19.3 Activities related to kilocalories

Activity	Time (min)	Kilocalories
Reading aloud	30	15
Washing dishes	15	19
Bicycle riding	60	150
Playing squash	60	916
Running	50	660
Walking	60	400

Microactivity and obesity

Microactivity describes minor, ostensibly trivial movements that occur within daily life: macroactivity describes the tasks a person performs composed of the sum of microactivity. A task can be performed using minimum energy expenditure, or embellished, depending on intensity of the microactivity underpinning it. It is estimated that sitting immobile utilises approximately $1\,\text{cal}\,\text{min}^{-1}$, whereas standing increases the calorie consumption by twofold and gentle strolling increases usage threefold. It is also suggested that to sustain weight previously lost requires a calorie deficit of around 150 per day. Therefore, something as simple as walking around while talking on the mobile phone rather than sitting at a desk, for, say, an hour a day can provide the extra deficit. Other examples of microactivity are 'fidgeting' movements of the legs, taking the stairs and even hand gesticulations during speech.

Lifestyle and obesity

Several major landmark studies have examined the effect of lifestyle interventions including physical activity on developing obesity-related diseases. A recent study from China assessed progression of IGT to type 2 diabetes mellitus in a Chinese population with three active treatment groups: diet alone; exercise alone; diet and exercise. The diet, exercise and diet-plus-exercise interventions resulted in 31%, 46% and 42% relative risk reduction for developing diabetes, respectively, whether or not individuals were overweight or lean. Furthermore, a 20-year follow-up showed that the relative risk reduction after early intensive lifestyle intervention is maintained in the long term, reflecting the findings of the United Kingdom Prospective Diabetes Study (UKPDS) 'legacy effect' in diabetes, whereby long-term protection against diabetic complications is conferred by early intensive treatment, regardless of the quality of management after the cessation of the trial. The Diabetes Prevention Programme compared lifestyle interventions and drug treatments on development of diabetes in a high-risk dysglycaemic population. Cumulative incidence of diabetes was reduced by an impressive 58% in those receiving lifestyle interventions at 4 years as a result of diet and physical activity even compared with metformin, a glucose-lowering agent; a powerful message that lifestyle not only has a role in the management of obese 'prediabetic' patients, but is an essential component. Interestingly, the Finnish Diabetes Prevention Study showed an identical 58% reduction in the cumulative incidence of diabetes as a result of lifestyle changes after 6 years.

The built environment and obesity

The National Institute for Health and Care Excellence (NICE) published guidelines on the built environments to help individuals become more physically active. As the built environment is identified as a major contributor to obesity, action is necessary to encourage individuals to use more energy. Planners, designers and architects have a responsibility to ensure that spaces and buildings offer their users the possibility of expending energy to maintain and improve health. People need to be more physically active, with better walking and cycling opportunities, and with building, offices and homes offering better access and signposting to stairs rather than lifts, and other active pursuits. An elegant study from the 1970s observed post office workers, demonstrating that those confined to sedentary desk jobs had a significantly greater risk of MI than those delivering letters.

Further reading

http://www.nhs.uk/Livewell/fitness/Pages/physical-activity-guidelines-for-adults.aspx
http://www.who.int/dietphysicalactivity/PA-promotionguide-2007.pdf?ua=1
http://www.who.int/dietphysicalactivity/end-childhood-obesity/en/
http://nutrition.org.uk/attachments/101_Physical%20activity%20and%20health.pdf
http://ukactive.com/downloads/managed/Turning_the_tide_of_inactivity.pdf

CHAPTER 20

Sport and Children

Neil Armstrong

Children's Health and Exercise Research Centre, University of Exeter, Exeter, UK

OVERVIEW

In this chapter we describe the area of children in sport. After studying this chapter, the reader will know

- The physical characteristics of the elite young athlete
- The effects of growth and maturation on youth sport performance
- The development of muscle strength, aerobic fitness and high intensity exercise performance during youth
- The effects of training and 'overtraining' during youth
- Relative age effects on youth sport

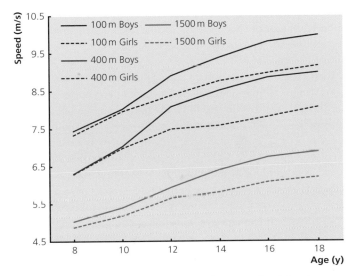

Figure 20.1 Average speed of world best performances in relation to age and sex. The 100 m sprint is supported by the catabolism of phosphocreatine and anaerobic glycolysis with ~10% of the energy being provided by aerobic metabolism. During youth, a 400 m sprint is ~60 to 70% supported by anaerobic metabolism, predominantly glycolysis, with minor support from aerobic sources. The 1500 m is a ~80% aerobic event although increases in pace (e.g. final sprint) have high anaerobic components

Elite young athletes in most sports experience several years of training and high-level competition during growth and maturation. It is not unusual to see children as young as 2 years of age in gymnastics induction programmes. Time engaged in training increases with age and elite gymnasts, and swimmers can spend ~30 h per week training during childhood. Participation in organised, competitive sport often begins as young as 6 to 7 years of age, and in gymnastics, for example, girls reach their competitive peak in their mid- to late-teens. Success in sport during youth is underpinned by a range of age-related and gender-related physical and physiological variables, which operate in a sport-specific manner and are dependent on the progress of individual 'biological clocks'. Performance asynchronously improves with age, growth and maturation, and there are marked gender differences. This is clearly illustrated by world best performances in relation to age and gender in athletic events primarily supported by different energy systems (Figure 20.1).

Physical characteristics of elite young athletes

Elite young athletes in most sports are generally taller than their non-athletic peers although in some sports height varies with playing position (e.g. soccer, basketball). Gymnastics is the only sport

in which both sexes consistently present a profile of below average height. Most elite young athletes have physiques and body shapes that promote their sport performance with young athletes in several sports (e.g. racquet sports, rowing, throwing events) being characterised by beneficial shoulder-to-hip and/or limb-to-trunk ratios. Elite young athletes typically have body weights that equal or exceed their chronological age-matched peers, and they are generally thinner than similar aged non-athletes, with the difference more pronounced in girls (Table 20.1).

Growth and maturation

All young people experience a similar pattern of growth and maturation, but there are wide individual variations in the magnitude of growth and in the timing of the initiation and rate of progress through puberty. The onset of girls' adolescent growth spurt occurs ~2 years earlier than that of boys, but growth during

---

ABC of Sports and Exercise Medicine, Fourth Edition.
Edited by Gregory P. Whyte, Mike Loosemore and Clyde Williams.
© 2015 John Wiley & Sons, Ltd. Published 2015 by John Wiley & Sons, Ltd.

Table 20.1 Heights and weights of young athletes relative to reference data percentiles (P)

Sport	Height		Weight	
	Males	Females	Males	Females
Basket ball	P50 to >P90	P75 to >P90	P50 to >P90	P50 to P75
Swimming	P50 to P90	P50 to P90	>P50 to P75	P50 to P75
Tennis	±P50	>P50	≥P50	±P50
Soccer	±P50	P50	±P50	P50
Sprints	≥P50	≥P50	≥P50	≤P50
Distance runs	±P50	≥P50	≤P50	<P50
Gymnastics	≤P10 to P25	≥P50	≤P10 to P25	P10 to <P50

Source: Adapted from Malina 1994, "Physical growth and biological maturation of young athletes". Reproduced by permission of Wolters Kluwer Health ONE EDN ONLY

puberty is characterised not only by increases in height but also by gender-specific body shape changes such as shoulder-to-hip and limb-to-trunk ratios.

Increases in boys' body mass during puberty are primarily due to gains in skeletal mass and muscle mass with percentage of fat mass declining from ~16% to ~12 to 14% of body mass. Muscle mass as a percentage of body mass increases from ~42% to 54% over the age range of 7 to 17, but peak muscle growth velocity is a relatively late event during puberty. During their growth spurt, girls experience a rise in percentage of fat mass from ~18% to 25% of body mass although values of ~14% have been noted in elite young gymnasts. Girls do not experience a similar spurt in muscle mass to boys and from age of 5 to 13 years girls' percentage of muscle mass increases from ~40% to 45% of their body mass and then in relative terms percentage of muscle mass declines due to a maturity-driven accumulation of fat.

Earlier maturing boys benefit from changes in body size, shape and composition, which are advantageous in most sports. For example, during puberty, boys experience an increase in limb length, a marked spurt in shoulder breadth, and an increase in muscle mass that is reflected by an increase in muscle strength. Even small differences in shoulder width can result in large differences in trunk muscle, and when this is combined with the greater leverage of longer arms the advantages of early maturity on performance in sports such as tennis and athletic throwing events is readily apparent. Since selection for youth sport is based on chronological age, few later maturing boys are successful during early adolescence except in sports such as gymnastics.

In youth sport, earlier maturing girls are less dominant than earlier maturing boys. Girls who mature early for their age have an advantage in sports that are reliant on body size but their wider hips, relatively shorter legs and greater body fatness are disadvantageous in some sports. Conversely, later-maturing girls present characteristics such as more linear physiques with lower weight-to-height ratios, less fatness, relatively longer legs and lower hip-to-shoulder ratios, which are more suitable for success in many sports. Age at menarche indicates a tendency for athletes to be later maturers, but most athletes fall within the normal range of variation. Only gymnasts consistently present average ages of menarche more than two standard deviations from the population mean but this is probably a result of selection and retention in the sport of later maturing

girls. There is no compelling evidence to suggest that growth, the initiation of puberty or the rate of progression through puberty is affected by intensive training or sport participation.

Muscle strength

Muscle strength increases almost linearly with chronological age from early childhood through to ~14 years when, in boys but not girls, there is a marked spurt through late adolescence, followed by a slower increase into young adulthood. Gender-related differences in muscle strength are small prior to puberty, and as girls enter puberty earlier than boys it is not unusual for 10 to 12-year-old girls to be stronger than similar aged boys. However, even after adjusting for body size differences, by late adolescence boys are significantly stronger than girls, particularly in the arms and trunk. In many sports, superior strength distinguishes the elite young athlete from the less successful performer and, therefore, earlier maturing boys have a significant advantage over their later maturing peers (Figure 20.2).

Supervised resistance training provides a safe and effective means of increasing muscle strength, and resistance training programmes are a key component of elite young athletes' overall training programmes. They should be initiated with moderate resistances followed by a gradual progression to greater resistances and fewer repetitions in accord with the individual's rate of growth and maturation. As elite young athletes gain experience, training programmes become individualised and more sport specific (Table 20.2).

The mechanisms underlying changes in muscle strength with training vary with age and maturation and possibly with gender. In pre-pubertal children, strength gains can be attributed primarily to neurological adaptations such as enhanced neural drive, increased motor unit synchronisation and reduced central nervous system inhibition. Muscle hypertrophy is the dominant influence during late adolescence, at least in boys. Resistance training induces similar (or greater) relative increases in muscle strength in children than in adolescents and adults but smaller absolute gains. There is no compelling evidence to suggest gender-related differences in responses

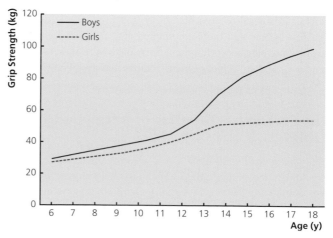

Figure 20.2 Muscle strength in relation to age and sex. Data from Malina et al., *Growth, Maturation and Physical Activity*

Table 20.2 Resistance training and muscle strength

- *Risks of injury*: resistance exercise is a safe and effective way of training and the injury risks are no greater than those associated with other well-supervised sports training programmes
- *Frequency*: two to three sessions per week (not consecutive days)
- *Intensity*: 8 to 15 repetitions at 60 to 80% of 1 repetition maximum (RM)[a]
- *Duration*: 3 sets of 6 to 8 exercises
- *Programme length*: 8 to 12 weeks
- *Expected gains*: ~10 to 40% with heterogeneity across muscle groups

[a]RM is the maximum number of repetitions that can be performed at a given resistance.
Source: Data from Armstrong and Van Mechelen, *Paediatric Exercise Science and Medicine*

to resistance training among pre- and early pubertal children although absolute muscle strength increases may be greater in boys during late adolescence.

Aerobic fitness

Peak oxygen uptake ($\dot{V}O_{2peak}$), the highest rate at which oxygen can be consumed during exercise, is recognised as the best single measure of aerobic fitness. There is an almost linear increase in boys' $\dot{V}O_{2peak}$ with age and a similar but less consistent trend in girls' values with a tendency to level-off at ~14 years. $\dot{V}O_{2peak}$ increases by ~150% in boys and ~80% in girls over the age range 8 to 16 years with the gender difference increasing from ~10% at age 10 to ~35% by age 16. As there are no gender differences in maximal heart rate (HR_{max}), the pre-pubertal gender difference in $\dot{V}O_{2peak}$ is primarily due to boys' greater maximal stroke index but whether this is caused by differences in cardiac size or cardiac function remains unknown. Increasing muscle mass is the dominant influence on $\dot{V}O_{2peak}$ during adolescence and accounts for much of the gender difference during the late teens, perhaps supplemented by boys' greater blood haemoglobin concentration. Maturation has a significant positive effect on $\dot{V}O_{2peak}$ independent of age, body size and body composition and gives those maturing earlier an advantage over individuals maturing later in sports influenced by aerobic fitness. $\dot{V}O_{2peak}$ is strongly correlated with body mass and when $\dot{V}O_{2peak}$ is scaled for body mass ($ml\,kg^{-1}\,min^{-1}$), a different picture emerges. Boys' mass-related $\dot{V}O_{2peak}$ remains essentially unchanged from 8 to 18 years at ~48 to 50 $ml\,kg^{-1}\,min^{-1}$, whereas girls' values reflect their relative increase in fat mass and decline from ~45 to 35 $ml\,kg^{-1}\,min^{-1}$ over the same period (Figure 20.3).

Elite young athletes present peak $\dot{V}O_{2peak}$ values ~30 to 50% higher than their non-athletic peers, but this is likely to be due to both selection and training. For training to induce significant gains in $\dot{V}O_{2peak}$ during youth, the relative intensity of the exercise needs to be within the HR range 170 to 180 beats per minute (85 to 90% of HR_{max}), which is higher than that which has been shown to be effective in adults. During childhood and adolescence, there are no age, maturational or gender effects on the magnitude of expected gains in $\dot{V}O_{2peak}$ with training but percentage changes tend to be less than those expected with adults. In both children and adults, the primary mechanism for training-induced changes in $\dot{V}O_{2peak}$ is enhanced delivery of oxygen to the muscles through

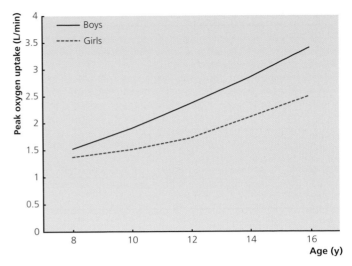

Figure 20.3 Peak oxygen uptake in relation to age and sex. Data from Armstrong and Van Mechelen, *Paediatric Exercise Science and Medicine*

Table 20.3 International Olympic Committee recommendations for enhancing the aerobic fitness (peak oxygen uptake) of the elite young athlete

- *Frequency of exercise*: 3 to 4 sessions each week
- *Duration of exercise*: 40 to 60 min each session
- *Intensity of exercise*: 85 to 90% of maximal heart rate
- *Expected gains*: ~5 to 10% increase in peak oxygen uptake in 8 to 12 weeks. There is no effect of sex or stage of maturation on expected gains but there is an estimated genetic effect of 40-50%

Source: Data from Armstrong and McManus, *The Elite Young Athlete*

an increase in stroke volume. There is a paucity of data on genetic influences on endurance training during youth, but it appears that, as with adults, there is a continuum from low responders to high responders (Table 20.3).

A high $\dot{V}O_{2peak}$ is a prerequisite for elite performance in several sports but in others the ability to engage in rapid changes in exercise intensity is paramount, and it is the transient kinetics of pulmonary $\dot{V}O_2$ that best describe the relevant component of aerobic fitness. The $\dot{V}O_2$ kinetics time constant can be used as a proxy measure of muscle phosphocreatine (PCr) kinetics and, therefore, as a non-invasive window into the metabolic activity of the muscle. Rigorously determined and analysed data on children's $\dot{V}O_2$ kinetic response to the onset of heavy and very heavy intensity exercise (> lactate threshold but < $\dot{V}O_{2peak}$) are sparse but show children's responses to be faster than those of adults. The $\dot{V}O_2$ kinetics response reflects muscle biopsy data and is consistent with the notion that children have an enhanced oxidative but attenuated anaerobic energy transfer during exercise compared with adults. No prospective studies have reported the effects of training on $\dot{V}O_2$ kinetics during youth but comparisons of girl swimmers with age-matched controls have demonstrated faster $\dot{V}O_2$ kinetics in the trained girls both before and during puberty (Table 20.4).

High-intensity exercise

The performance of brief high-intensity exercise primarily supported by anaerobic energy sources is central to most sports

Table 20.4 Pulmonary oxygen uptake kinetics

- Many sports are dependent on repeated, rapid changes in exercise intensity, and under these conditions pulmonary $\dot{V}O_2$ kinetics rather than peak $\dot{V}O_2$ is the primary component
- No relationships between the $p\dot{V}O_2$ kinetic time constant and peak$\dot{V}O_2$ have been demonstrated in either trained or untrained youth
- Children have faster $p\dot{V}O_2$ kinetic responses than adults and boys have faster $p\dot{V}O_2$ kinetic responses than girls during the transition from rest or low intensity exercise to heavy exercise
- Training-induced speeding of $p\dot{V}O_2$ kinetics might enhance performance by resisting fatigue
- Faster $p\dot{V}O_2$ kinetic responses to the onset of heavy exercise have been demonstrated in trained groups of both pre-pubertal and pubertal girl swimmers compared with age-matched controls

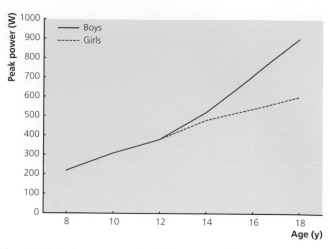

Figure 20.4 Peak power output in relation to age and sex. Data from Armstrong et al., "Short term power output in relation to growth and maturation" and Van Praagh, "Development of anaerobic function during childhood and adolescence"

(e.g. soccer, rugby, sprints [100 to 400 m]), but direct analysis of the underlying muscle energetics is limited by ethical restrictions on the use of invasive techniques with healthy children. In the absence of intra-muscle data, paediatric research has focused on the assessment of external power output and variants of the Wingate anaerobic test (WAnT) have emerged as the most popular tests of young people's power output. The WAnT allows the determination of peak power (PP) usually over a 1-, 3- or 5-second period and mean power (MP) over the 30 s test period. There is an almost linear increase in PP and MP in both genders from ~7 to 13 years, and then boys demonstrate a second and steeper increase in power output through to young adulthood. Prior to the male spurt in power output, girls often outscore boys of the same age as a result of their more advanced maturation, but by the age of 18 years the gender difference in PP is ~50%. From 12 to 17 years, boys increase their PP by ~120% and their MP by ~110% compared with girls who increase their PP by ~66% and their MP by ~60%. The asynchronous development of the anaerobic and aerobic energy systems is illustrated by increases in aerobic power ($\dot{V}O_{2peak}$) over the same age range being ~70% and ~25% in boys and girls, respectively. This difference in anaerobic and aerobic development is clearly reflected in world age group records (Figure 20.4).

Compared with the extant data on training-induced changes in muscle strength and $\dot{V}O_{2peak}$, few data on the effects of high-intensity training on power output have been reported. Furthermore, non-specific training of brief high-intensity activities on target muscles is difficult to quantify with the criterion tests available. The weight of evidence suggests that muscle power gains during youth are in the range 5 to 12% following a 12-week training programme, but data are insufficient to warrant comment on the influence of age, maturation or gender. The few muscle biopsy data available from boys indicate increases in adenosine triphosphate, PCr and glycogen concentrations in the resting muscle following training. There are no similar data from girls.

Unexplained underperformance syndrome

The effects of training programmes during youth are generally beneficial, but recent surveys suggest that unexplained underperformance syndrome (UPS) is experienced by ~30% of elite young athletes. UPS is more prevalent in individual sports (~37%) than in

Table 20.5 Unexplained underperformance syndrome (UPS)

Symptoms

- Underperformance and increased fatigue
- Increased perception of effort during exercise
- Raised resting heart rate
- Frequent upper respiratory tract infections
- Muscle soreness
- Sleep disturbances
- Loss of appetite
- Mood disorders
- Shortness of temper and/or conflicts with coach and family
- Decreased self-confidence
- Depression
- Decreased interest in training and competition
- Inability to concentrate

Treatment/management

- Cross-training (introduce fun into sessions)
- Light-to-moderate aerobic exercise
- Skill practice
- Massage
- Hydrotherapy
- Counselled relaxation sessions
- Gradual re-introduction to training and competition

UPS occurs where high-intensity training, frequent competition and non-sport-specific stressors combine to negatively affect the young athlete.

team sports (~17%) and in girls (~36%) more than boys (~26%). Very high training loads and intense, frequent competitions provide the primary underlying cause of UPS, but UPS in elite young athletes may be even more multidimensional than in adults. For example, the stress caused by the developmental and peer-group pressures of adolescence, the loss of autonomy in lifestyle planning through devotion to a single sporting goal, coping with the combined demands of school, examinations, training and competition, and striving to manage the often unrealistic expectations of coaches and parents contribute to UPS during youth (Table 20.5).

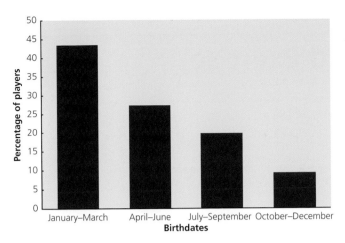

Figure 20.5 Birth date distribution in relation to selection year – the relative age effect. Birth dates of the U15, U16, U17 and U18 national soccer teams from 10 European countries. Data from Helsen *et al.*, "The relative age effect in youth soccer across Europe"

Selection, retention and the relative age effect

Growth and maturation are important components of both selection and retention in youth sport. As individuals born near the beginning of the selection year are likely to be more biologically mature than those born almost a year later, birth date strongly influences the chances of success in elite youth sport. The most well-documented example of this is the relative age effect in youth soccer although it has also been demonstrated in numerous sports including tennis, swimming, rugby and ice hockey. For example, the birth date distribution in relation to the selection year (1 January to 31 December) of the U15, U16, U17 and U18 national soccer teams of 10 European countries demonstrates, both by country and combined, statistically significant differences with 43% of the players born in the first quarter and 9% born in the last quarter of the selection year. Unequal birth date distribution persists into the senior game in which almost 40% of English Premier League footballers were born in the first quarter of the youth selection year (Figure 20.5).

Future research directions

Research with children presents many challenges and much remains to be learnt about physiological responses to exercise in relation to age, growth and maturation. Recently, techniques initially pioneered with adults and non-invasive technologies have been successfully modified for use with children. New experimental models have been developed and together these innovations have opened up intriguing new avenues for future research in developmental physiology with reference to identifying, selecting and nurturing elite young athletes (Table 20.6).

Sport and well-being

Many young people achieve success in sport but some talented youngsters are denied access to elite youth sport, and potentially

Table 20.6 Future research directions

- To apply non-invasive technology (e.g. magnetic resonance spectroscopy, near-infra red spectroscopy, breath-by-breath respiratory gas analysis) and innovative experimental models (e.g. priming exercise, work-to-work transitions, manipulation of components of exercise intensity) to the development of greater understanding of exercise metabolism during growth and maturation
- To develop valid field and laboratory tests with the necessary specificity for confident monitoring of sports performance during youth
- To determine the immediate and future positive and negative effects of long-term aerobic, resistance and high-intensity training during childhood and adolescence
- To examine the incidence, causes and treatment of UPS in young athletes
- To seek solution(s) to the relative age effect in youth sport

to elite adult sport, through selection policies which are driven by factors related to growth and maturation. Other children and adolescents drop-out prematurely through ill-advised early specialisation in sports, which turn out to be inappropriate for their late adolescent physiology or physique. Adults working with children should focus on fostering participation in sport for all, identifying talent, and nurturing it irrespective of the ticking of individual biological clocks.

> ADULTS INVOLVED IN YOUTH SPORT SHOULD FOCUS ON THE ROLE OF SPORT IN PROMOTING THE HEALTH AND WELL-BEING OF THE CHILD, AND NOT ON THE ROLE OF THE CHILD IN PROMOTING THE HEALTH AND WELL-BEING OF SPORT

Further reading

Armstrong, N. & McManus, A.M. (eds) (2011) *The Elite Young Athlete*. Karger, Basle.

Armstrong N, Van Mechelen W. (eds) (2008) *Paediatric Exercise Science and Medicine* (2nd ed.). Oxford University Press, Oxford.

Armstrong, N., Welsman, J.R. & Chia, M.Y.H. (2005) Short term power output in relation to growth and maturation. *British Journal of Sports Medicine*, **35**, 118–124.

Hebestreit, H. & Bar-Or, O. (eds) (2008) *The Young Athlete*. Blackwell, Oxford.

Helsen, W.F., Van Winckel, J. & Williams, M. (2005) The relative age effect in youth soccer across Europe. *Journal of Sports Sciences*, **23**, 629–636.

Malina, R.M. (1994) Physical growth and biological maturation of young athletes. *Exercise and Sport Sciences Reviews*, **22**, 389–433.

Malina, R.M., Bouchard, C. & Bar-Or, O. (2004) *Growth, Maturation and Physical Activity*, 2nd edn. Human Kinetics, Champaign, IL.

Malina, R.M., Baxter-Jones, A.D.G., Armstrong, N. *et al.* (2013) Role of intensive training on growth and maturation in artistic gymnastics. *Sports Medicine*, **43**, 783–802.

Van Praagh, E. (2000) Development of anaerobic function during childhood and adolescence. *Pediatric Exercise Science*, **12**, 150–173.

CHAPTER 21

Physical Activity and Exercise in Later Life

Dawn A. Skelton[1] and Finbarr C. Martin[2]

[1]School of Health and Life Sciences, Institute of Applied Health Research, Glasgow Caledonian University, Glasgow, UK
[2]Guys & St Thomas' NHS Foundation Trust, London, UK, Westminster Bridge Road, London, UK

OVERVIEW

- A physically active lifestyle enhances independent living no matter what a person's age or fitness
- Avoidance of sedentary behaviour is increasingly considered to be as important as promotion of physical activity
- Many older people lack confidence to participate, and have off putting misconceptions about the benefits and risks
- Exercise interventions can improve quality of life, physical and psychological health in older people with a range of medical conditions and functional abilities
- Encouragement and motivation to be more active has a key place in the medical practitioners toolbox
- Those older people with more complex conditions should be referred to trained specialists for improved outcomes, effectiveness and safety

---

Regular physical activity and exercise improves physiological and psychological outcomes

Evidence for the benefits of physical activity promotion and exercise interventions with older people is overwhelming (Box 21.1), and now the focus rests on strategies to increase uptake and adherence to long-term active lifestyles and to apply the evidence-based interventions for specific indications. Many government and clinical guidelines now exist to encourage practitioners and professionals to promote physical activity and exercise for older people. There are recommendations for brief advice in primary care and advice on motivation and behavioural strategies to help motivate people to be more active. Specific guidance exists about exercise interventions for falls and the prevention of frailty and functional decline. This supported by guidance on exercise referral systems.

Prevention and management of disease

Regular physical activity throughout the lifespan helps prevent conditions that are more common in old age, including osteoporosis,

---

Box 21.1 Definitions of physical activity and exercise

Physical activity is defined as any bodily movement produced by skeletal muscles that results in energy expenditure.

Exercise is a subset of physical activity that is planned, structured, and repetitive and has as a final or an intermediate objective the improvement or maintenance of physical fitness.

Source: Caspersen *et al.* (1985)

---

non-insulin-dependent diabetes mellitus, hypertension, ischaemic heart disease, stroke and many cancers (Figure 21.1). Even in old age, maintaining or increasing activity is vital for the preservation of function and reduction of symptoms in the presence of disease. Exercise interventions aimed at improving specific components of fitness, as opposed to increasing physical activity, are the mainstay of cardiac, pulmonary, stroke, cancer and falls rehabilitation programmes.

Prevention of disability, frailty and immobility

Not only does regular physical activity play an important part in preventing or managing symptoms of disease, it can help prevent dependency (Box 21.2). Key to this is maintaining individuals'

Box 21.2 Psychological benefits of physical activity and exercise

Regular physical activity	Exercise interventions
Improved sleep duration and quality	Reduced fear of falling
Improved mental health	Improved sleep duration and quality
Improved vitality	Improved cognitive speed
Improved autonomy	Improved auditory and visual attention
Improved mood	Improved confidence
Reduced depression	Improved executive functioning

Source: Montgomery and Dennis (2002), Angevaren *et al.* (2008), Liu Ambrose *et al.* (2008), NICE (2013), Kendrick *et al.* (2014), Vagetti *et al.* (2014).

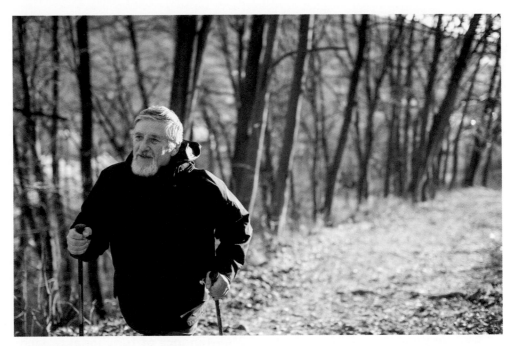

Figure 21.1 Nordic walking is a popular form of fitness walking. Source: Bigstock Photos #62178413. Reproduced with permission

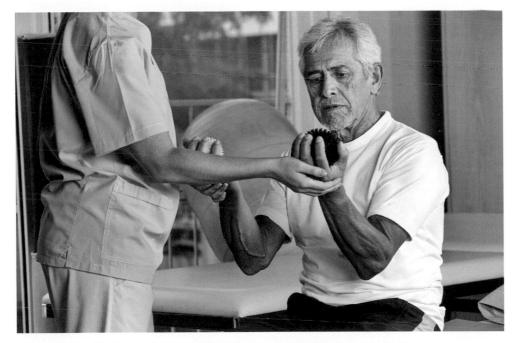

Figure 21.2 Frailer older people require skilled instruction. Source: Bigstock Photos # 42291376. Reproduced with permission

strength, stamina and balance above threshold levels for functional ability (Figure 21.2). Even the frailest, oldest adult will benefit from graded exercise training to maintain or improve function. Sarcopenia and frailty are common in people who avoid activity either as a result of concern about their condition or for fear of falling; therefore, strategies to increase participation in regular activity and to maintain muscle strength should be considered as part of all medical consultations.

Even those who are disabled to the extent they cannot weight bear independently benefit from seated exercise and movement that stimulates circulation, just as passengers sitting on long plane journeys benefit. The prevention of faecal impaction, reduced risk of deep vein thrombosis and gravitational oedema are all prevented or managed with regular movement.

From about the age of 30–40 we are all ageing in terms of declining strength, power (speed with which we can use muscle strength), balance and flexibility, stamina and co-ordination. But the rate of change is highly variable, reflecting genetic, early life experiences and later lifestyle patterns, as well as cumulative effects of multimorbidity. Muscle power declines earlier and more precipitously than muscle strength, and is a more important predictor of functional limitations in older adults

As everyday tasks become more difficult, or are perceived to be more effortful, most people adapt by modifying or avoiding these activities and so the spiral of decline of physical performance through inactivity is additive to the effects of ageing. Fear of falling, irrespective of having fallen, is a risk factor for both future falls and activity limitation, with a resulting spiralling risk of functional decline and, as such, is an early indicator of mobility impairment and a target for preventative action.

Breathlessness on walking is often not a function of disease, but lack of fitness such that even slow walking is requiring a large percentage of the individual's maximal aerobic capacity.

A body of epidemiological evidence exists, suggesting that inactivity (not meeting the physical activity guidelines) is one of the major causes of functional decline. Sedentary behaviour (sitting, reclining or lying down in the waking day) (Box 21.3) is a pattern of behaviour distinct from inactivity and its effects on health are noticeable even if people reach physical activity recommendations (Box 21.3).

Sedentary behaviour has been linked to frailty, mortality and chronic health problems, and is also likely to affect function, quality of life and social inclusion. Older adults are the most sedentary sector of the population, spending on average 80% of their waking day (8–12 h) in sedentary activities so it is important that all health professionals encourage regular sit to stand transitions to break up prolonged periods of sitting (Box 21.4).

In hospitalised patients

Patients in hospital are particularly sedentary. On average, patients are in an upright position for only 70 ($\pm$50) minutes per day, with 70% of this time spent in standing or walking epochs of less than 5 min. Lower limb strength is important, not just to ensure people

> Box 21.3 **Sedentary behaviour definition**
>
> Any waking activity characterised by an energy expenditure $\leq$ 1.5 METs, and a sitting or reclining posture.
>
> Source: Sedentary Behaviour Network (2012)

> Box 21.4 **Effects of sedentary behaviour in old age**
>
> Those who sit for prolonged periods in their day, compared to those that do not:
>
> - Twice as likely to have high blood pressure, high cholesterol and metabolic syndrome
> - Four times as likely to have a high waist: hip ratio
> - Higher risk of osteoporosis and musculoskeletal pain
> - Lower quality of life and levels of social inclusion and engagement
>
> Each additional hour of TV watching a day is associated with a 19% increased likelihood of metabolic syndrome.

can transfer easily, but to live independently and help maintain core temperature. There is also a strong relationship between chair rise ability (use of hands to rise) and all-cause mortality (taking into account age, body mass index and gender). Accordingly, patients should be encouraged to get up every hour they have sat, this alone will contribute to improved strength outcomes by increasing the number of weight transfers each day. Multidisciplinary intervention that includes exercise increases the proportion of patients discharged home and reduces length and cost of hospital stay for acutely hospitalised older medical patients.

Inactivity is one of the many risk factors for falls. Another concern for increased falls risk is recent research, suggesting that older people sitting in a cold room (15 °C) for just 45 min can lead to a loss of muscle power in the region of 5%, a 10% reduction in sit to stand speed, reduced quadriceps strength and slower walking speed. Similarly, sitting for 45 min in a hot room (30 °C) for the same amount of time can also have potential falls risk effects by reducing blood pressure and walking speed, and increasing the risk of orthostatic hypotension.

Maintenance of functional capacity

Regular exercise increases strength, power, balance, co-ordination, endurance and flexibility. Even those over the age of 75 can rejuvenate 20 years of lost strength in a 12-week progressive programme. In percentage terms, the improvements seen in older people are similar to those seen in younger people. Exercise programmes with differing foci on specific components of fitness are effective at improving function and quality of life after stroke and aerobic capacity in heart failure (particularly endurance work). Progressive strength and balance training (for an effective dose of about 50 h) is effective at reducing falls, and sarcopenia can be improved with programmes focusing on nutrition and strength, with effectiveness equal to that seen in younger adults. Increased activity, performed regularly, improves sleep patterns, reduces arthritic pain, can help improve the pelvic floor muscles and therefore facilitate social participation, improve continence and reduce isolation. Mobility training is effective even in the frailest older adults.

Prevention of isolation

In addition to the physiological improvements, physical activity and exercise offer important opportunities for socialisation. It also permits the emotional benefits of socially acceptable touching, unconnected with dependence and the need for personal care. Touching is a rarity for many older people who are long bereaved. Much research has focused on the psychologically beneficial effects of group exercise, in terms of peer support, feeling part of a group, increased activity outwith the class environment by group members and reduced anxiety, depression and fear of falling. Having the energy and capacity to 'do what you want to do when you want to do it' are important outcomes of a physically active lifestyle.

Providing advice and opportunity

What type of activity?

To help maintain function and health, physical activity advice should focus on ensuring that the individual has a varied menu of

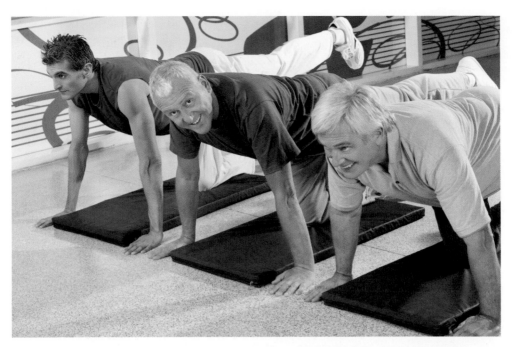

Figure 21.3 Floorwork is important to reduce fear of falling. Source: Bigstock Photos #31718087. Reproduced with permission

options that will continue to challenge all the main components of fitness. Any exercise programme to improve fitness in older people should include all components of fitness that are core to good functional capacity, such as endurance, flexibility, strength, power, balance and co-ordination, in a tailored and progressive way. The type of activities that older people choose will often reflect their personal history, likes and dislikes. Many older people walk or have walked a lot in the past and this is a good place to start, but walking is not enough to significantly improve strength and balance and unless done briskly is unlikely to improve endurance or bone health. In fact, brisk walking alone as an intervention may be unsafe and is not recommended for those with a history of falls as risk may be increased due to poor balance worsened by fatigue.

Many will enjoy swimming or cycling, but it is important to consider if the activities consist of an adequate variety of the components of fitness necessary to maintain independence: it is often strengthening and balance activities that are omitted. Muscle strength work should focus on major muscle groups in exercises that train through the fullest pain free range of movement. A well-programmed general fitness session also aims to load the bones, train pelvic floor and postural muscles, practice functional movements and enhance body awareness and balance skills (Figure 21.3).

Strengthening activities can be anything that uses the body weight or extra resistance, for example, repeated slow sit to stands or use of ankle weights or resistance bands, which are performed to an intensity that the person 'feels the muscles' getting warmer, perhaps a bit wobbly and the next day they feel they have exercised them (Figure 21.4). In this way, they know that the exercise is providing a training effect. Balance challenging exercise can be anything from dancing or Tai Chi to standing on one leg next to the kitchen counter (Figure 21.5).

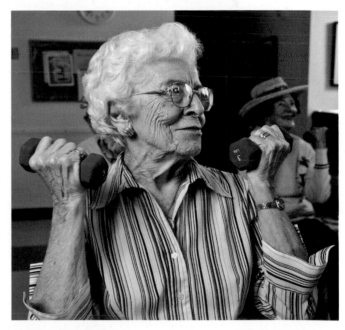

Figure 21.4 Strength training is important to prevent sarcopenia. Source: iStock # 000010210903. Reproduced with permission from iStockphoto.com

How much is enough?

The four Chief Medical Officer's (CMOs) (UK) have published guidelines on physical activity for health, specific to older people. Moderate intensity activity, which leads to the person feeling 'comfortably challenged, warmer than usual, and slightly breathless' (but can still hold a conversation), will vary for different people depending on their fitness and medical conditions but should be encouraged as often older people avoid activities that make them breathless and their heart beat faster and need to understand the

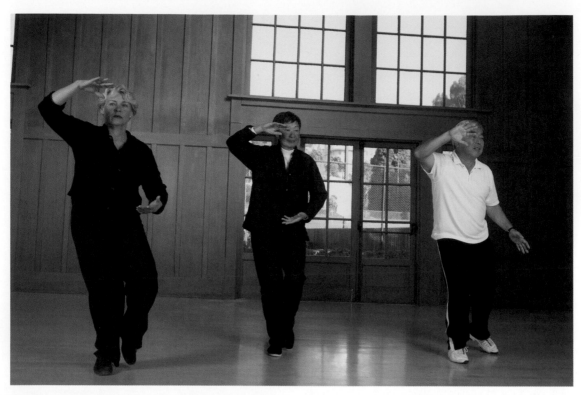

Figure 21.5 Tai Chi trains balance and lower limb strength. Source: Bigstock Photos #12054425. Reproduced with permission

---

> **Box 21.5 UK Physical Activity Guidelines – weekly recommendations for older people**
>
> - At least 150 min of moderate-intensity aerobic activity, or at least 75 min of vigorous-intensity aerobic activity, or an equivalent combination.
> - Aerobic activity should be performed in bouts of at least 10 min duration.
> - For additional health benefits, undertake up to 300 min of moderate-intensity or 150 min of vigorous-intensity aerobic activity, or an equivalent combination.
> - Those at risk of falls should do balance exercise on 2 or more days.
> - Muscle-strengthening activities should be done on 2 or more days.
> - Avoid prolonged periods of sitting in the day.
> - If older adults are unable to do the recommended amounts of physical activity due to health conditions, they should be as physically active as they are able.
>
> Source: Department of Health (2011)

value of such efforts. The CMOs also highlighted the need to avoid prolonged periods of sitting and adding activities that improve strength and challenge balance at least twice weekly (Box 21.5). For independently active older people, more vigorous activities are recommended but, of course, for frailer older people, being active every day and if referred to exercise, being supervised and guided by a specialist instructor is vital to promote independence. Even those people who are essentially chair or bed bound benefit from activity to promote circulation and regular practice and training in transfer skills to avoid risks of deep vein thrombosis, constipation and falls. An obstacle to participation is the mistaken belief by many frail patients that their habitual activity levels are adequate and that more would be detrimental to their recovery from illness.

Exercise groups or exercising alone

Although there are many effective home exercise programmes, particularly in falls prevention, motivation to adhere to home-based exercise without continued support and progression is often lacking and therefore people discontinue. Group exercise often fosters a feeling of group cohesion, peer support, new friends and an element of friendly competition that means effectiveness, adherence over time and progression is more assured (Figure 21.6). The role of a well-trained exercise instructor in fostering such group cohesion, self-efficacy and motivation are well known. When instructors deliver in a more motivational and enthusiastic manner, there are higher levels of participant enjoyment and adherence. Training and the context of exercise provision can enhance these important trainer qualities. Older adults may be worried about hurting themselves when exercising, and they feel more confident if they know that the instructor is adequately trained.

Safety

Injury prevention is a high priority. Even stiffness and minor overuse injuries reduce enjoyment and adherence. For the exercise instructor with an older adult qualification, the provision of an adequate warm-up, selection of safe exercises and movement patterns, regular monitoring of postural alignment, tailored progression of

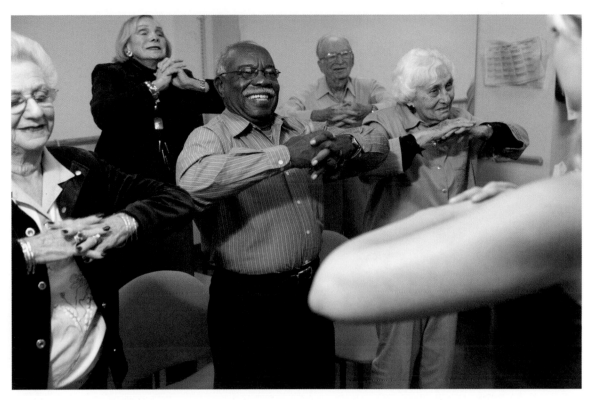

Figure 21.6 Group exercise aids motivation and adherence. Source: Bigstock Photos # 27574373. Reproduced with permission

exercise intensity and an appropriate warm down and stretch are all mainstays of a good session. Skilled demonstrations, observation and correction and class management are key to ensure safety. For those embarking on exercise and activity alone, starting slowly, progressing cautiously and listening to your body are the safest way to see improvements without injury. Falls are the most common adverse event reported in Cochrane Reviews of evidence about exercise for people with a variety of medical conditions, with the exception of exercise aimed at preventing falls! Therefore, particular attention to consideration of support options, graded progression of difficulty and avoidance of excessive fatigue are paramount. One-to-one rehabilitation from physiotherapists/exercise specialists and group sessions delivered by instructors with specialist qualifications (i.e. Level 4 on the Register of Exercise Professionals) exist to ensure that older people with a variety of different medical conditions are safely and effectively progressed through effective interventions.

Medical role

Primary care practitioners have been called to action in the 2013 NICE guidelines for brief advice to promote physical activity among all patients (Box 21.6).

Older adults, particularly those with chronic health conditions, have relatively high rates of attendance at their GP; this provides an opportunity for exercise-related advice. Older adults who received advice from their physician performed more moderate-to-vigorous intensity activity than those who did not. Giving specific physical activity advice, a plan of action and some form of follow-up are important factors in facilitating the uptake and maintenance of

Box 21.6 **NICE recommendations for promoting physical activity**

- identifying adults who are inactive
- delivering brief advice
- following up brief advice
- incorporating brief advice in commissioning
- systems to support brief advice
- information and training to support brief advice

Source: NICE (2013)

exercise programmes in older adults; this has been demonstrated in both physical activity programmes and exercise interventions. Furthermore, doctors should encourage other healthcare team members to support this approach, with skills and knowledge to identify obstacles and increase motivation. Guidance is available specifically addressing the needs of older people (Box 21.7).

What to advise, and to whom?

While there is no definitive evidence for a comprehensive model for all older populations of patients, there is sufficient evidence to apply a mix of general preventative approaches for all with more specific interventions for some. Physical activity should be considered as part of the management of any long-term condition, such as Chronic Obstructive Pulmonary Disease (COPD) or diabetes, but this advice should now be added to the identification and management of frailty. Consensus advice has been developed by

Box 21.7 **Medical referral responsibilities**

In making an exercise referral, the doctor has several responsibilities:

- To assess the individual's readiness to embark on a change in activity or exercise and apply brief motivational interventions as indicated.
- To discuss concerns such as embarrassment, safety and practicalities of participation.
- To agree with the patient a referral based on specific health-related objectives with achievable gains incorporated into an individualised plan, and arrange review of progress.
- To identify relevant medical conditions and ensure that all medications are communicated accurately to the exercise service, and to highlight any ways that the safe conduct of exercise might be influenced by these conditions (e.g. susceptibility to angina, shortness of breath, arrhythmias, joint pain and confusion) or by the medications (e.g. suppressing pain, producing a bradycardia unrepresentative of exercise intensity or increasing susceptibility to postural hypotension).
- To optimise treatment of any exercise-limiting conditions, bearing in mind that patients may have normalised their symptomatic limitations and not declare them.
- To educate the person exercising to recognise early symptoms that might indicate the exercise programme is, in some way, unsuitable for them (e.g. to recognise and respect an increase in pain, stiffness or swelling associated with osteoarthritis). But it is also necessary to emphasize that some symptoms are normal; for example, the patient with a history of controlled heart failure should be advised that increased breathing during exercise is normal but that a decrease in the level of exercise required to provoke shortness of breath is abnormal.

Source: Department of Health (2001)

a partnership of geriatricians, GPs, therapists, nurses and AgeUK to operationalise this in community settings (British Geriatrics Society).

Slow gait speed is one of several recommended frailty assessments and is a predictor of incident disability. Self-reported walking speed is a reasonable indication. This may be a good starting point for identifying early functional change and discussing better responses through increasing physical activity, rather than the maladaptive response of activity limitation.

Notwithstanding the challenges in achieving uptake and adherence, a review built on 20 randomised controlled trials that included 1378 participants showed consistent evidence that intensive physical rehabilitation enhances mobility and, when administered over a long period, may also improve the physical functioning of patients with dementia.

Most doctors in general or specialist practice will be less able than the trained exercise instructor to advise on the individualised prescription of particular exercises or activities, but can nevertheless play a vital role. Responsibility for the administration, design and delivery of the programme rests with the leisure management and instructor team or the exercise practitioner service, or both. The referring doctor should be assured (e.g. through commissioning) that those supervising the conduct of the exercise can demonstrate appropriate training and continuing professional development.

Acknowledgements

This chapter builds on a previous chapter edition written by Professor Archie Young (retired) and Dr Susie Dinan (retired) in 2005. Their original work, research and renown in the field are acknowledged as the building blocks of this updated chapter.

Conflicts of interest

DS is a Director of Later Life Training.

Further reading

British Geriatric Society Best Practice Guide. *Physical activity in older age*, BGS Website, 2010. Available from http://www.bgs.org.uk/index.php/topresources/publicationfind/goodpractice/1116-bpgphysicalactivity [accessed January 2015]

British Geriatrics Society. *Fit for frailty parts I & II*. http://www.bgs.org.uk/index.php/fitforfrailty-2m [accessed January 2015]

British Heart Foundation National Centre for Physical Activity and Health. *Interpreting the physical activity guidelines for older adults and other resources.* Available from http://www.bhfactive.org.uk/older-adults-resources-and-publications-results/39/index.html [accessed January 2015].

Clegg, A., Young, J., Iliffe, S., Rikkert, M.O. & Rockwood, K. (2013) Frailty in elderly people. *Lancet*, **381** (**9868**), 752–762.

Department of Health. *Start Active, Stay Active: A Report on Physical Activity for Health from the Four Home Countries' Chief Medical Officers.* Department of Health, Physical Activity, Health Improvement and Protection, London, 2011. Available from https://www.gov.uk/government/publications/start-active-stay-active-a-report-on-physical-activity-from-the-four-home-countries-chief-medical-officers [accessed January 2015]

Dinan, S. (2001) Exercise for vulnerable older patients. In: Young, A. & Harries, M. (eds), *Exercise Prescription for Patients.* Royal College of Physicians of London, London.

NICE. *PH44: Physical Activity: Brief Advice for Adults in Primary Care.* National Institute of Clinical Excellence, 2013. Available from: https://www.nice.org.uk/guidance/ph44 [accessed January 2015]

Nelson, M.E., Rejeski, W.J., Blair, S.N. *et al.* (2007) Physical activity and public health in older adults: recommendation from the American College of Sports Medicine and the American Heart Association. *Medicine and Science in Sports and Exercise*, **39** (**8**), 1435–1445.

Owen, N., Bauman, A. & Brown, W. (2009) Too much sitting: a novel and important predictor of chronic disease risk? *British Journal of Sports Medicine*, **43**, 81–83.

CHAPTER 22

Nutrition, Energy Metabolism and Ergogenic Supplements

Clyde Williams

School of Sport, Exercise and Health Sciences, Loughborough University, Loughborough, UK

OVERVIEW

- Role of nutrition for health and sport
- Importance of understanding principles of energy balance
- Essentials of energy metabolism during exercise
- Nutritional strategies for training and competition
- Supplements: types and functions

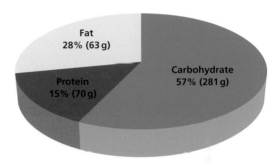

Figure 22.1 Composition of food intake of female distance runners (*n*=58) with a daily energy intake of 2000 kcal

Introduction

The role of nutrition in supporting training and competition is now well accepted. Nevertheless, one of the persistent myths is that there are 'ergogenic supplements' that, when found, will allow athletes to train hard, recover quickly and compete more successfully than their rivals. Searching for such 'quick-fix supplements' overshadows the important and essential contributions of commonly available foods to health and exercise performance. The first and foremost nutritional need of athletes is for a well-balanced diet, made up of a wide range of foods in sufficient quantity to cover their energy expenditure. Thereafter, they should adopt nutritional strategies to ensure that they can train, compete and recover more successfully than they would if left to follow their own appetites and perceptions of effective diets.

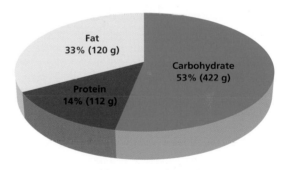

Figure 22.2 Composition of food intake of male distance runners (*n*=55) with a daily energy intake of 3220 kcal

Nutrition

Health professionals recommend that we eat a diet that contains a wide range of foods containing about 50% of energy from carbohydrate (CHO), about 15% from protein and the remainder from fat (avoiding large amounts of saturated fat). Endurance athletes have diets that generally match this recommendation for healthy eating (Figures 22.1 and 22.2). The daily energy intake of these female distance runners was about 2000 kcal, whereas the energy intake for this sample of male distance runners was 3220 kcal. However, even though endurance athletes have diets with similar proportions of

macronutrients, the quantities of food eaten are significantly different (Figures 22.1 and 22.2). Both groups of athletes maintain low body weights to avoid the detrimental impact on the performance of increased body mass. This is particularly true in female endurance athletes who have a daily energy intake that is not that different to the public at large, that is, 2000 kcal per day: they maintain a low body weight and cover up to 100 miles per week in training by consuming diets that are high in carbohydrate and very low in fat (Figure 22.1).

Macronutrients

Carbohydrate. Bread, potatoes, rice and pasta are the common forms of carbohydrates in our habitual diets. Other contributors are root vegetables such as parsnips, turnips, swedes, carrots and

ABC of Sports and Exercise Medicine, Fourth Edition.
Edited by Gregory P. Whyte, Mike Loosemore and Clyde Williams.
© 2015 John Wiley & Sons, Ltd. Published 2015 by John Wiley & Sons, Ltd.

Table 22.1 Glycaemic index

High	Moderate	Low
Glucose	Whole grain bread	Fructose
Sucrose	Spaghetti (pasta)	Yogurt
Cane	Corn	Peanuts
Maple syrup	Oatmeal	Peas
Corn syrup	Orange	Beans
Honey	Grapes	Apple
Corn flakes		Peach
Raisins		Pear
White rice		Figs
White bread		Milk

beetroot as well as fruit such as bananas, apples and pears. In the past, carbohydrates were regarded as either simple or complex. However, they are now more usefully classified in terms of the rise in blood glucose following the ingestion of a standard amount of carbohydrate (50 g) in relation to the glycaemic response to the same amount of glucose. Thus, carbohydrates are described as high glycaemic index (HGI) or low glycaemic index (LGI) depending on their glycaemic responses (Table 22.1). The LGI carbohydrates have high fibre content, and so their digestion and absorption are slower than low-fibre carbohydrates (HGI). After consuming LGI carbohydrates, the rise in plasma insulin is less than after consuming simple carbohydrates (HGI): consequently, the depression of fat mobilisation and metabolism is significantly less.

Protein. Although the recommended daily protein intake for the general public is $0.8\,g\,kg^{-1}$ body weight, it is the minimum amount needed to maintain health of adults. However, it is too low for children, pregnant women and athletes. The optimum amount for active individuals and athletes is between 1.5 and $1.8\,g\,kg^{-1}$ per day. High biological value proteins, such as meat, fish and eggs, contain all the essential amino acids that we need to build the body's vast range of proteins. The 8 essential amino acids must be obtained from our diet, whereas the remaining 12 amino acids can be synthesised within the body when not obtained by the diet. For most people, the evening meal provides most of our daily protein. However, in order to achieve optimum assimilation, athletes should spread out their daily protein intake across all meals including snacks.

Fat. Fat is stored in adipose tissue cells as triglycerides and is distributed subcutaneously and deep within the body. Some fat is also stored in skeletal muscles as droplets of triglycerides. Not all dietary fats constitute a health risk by, for example, increasing plasma cholesterol. Fats in oily fish such as sardines, mackerel and salmon have health benefits. These omega-3′fatty acids are, for example, incorporated into the membranes around nerve fibres as well as being an essential part of other tissues. In addition to being a concentrated source of energy, fats also provide us with the fat-soluble vitamins A, D, E and K.

Micronutrients

Vitamins and minerals are essential 'oils' that keep our metabolic machinery working effectively. They are required in only micro-amounts and are provided by a diet made up of a wide range of foods that are sufficient in quantity to support our daily activities. Those who are most at-risk of micronutrient insufficiency are athletes who under eat to achieve and maintain a lower than normal body weight to compete in lower weight categories or to improve their power-to-weight ratio.

Energy balance

When the energy we gain from our diet matches our energy expenditure, we are in energy balance and is reflected by a stable body weight. An energy intake that exceeds expenditure results in the excess being stored as fat and carbohydrate. Conversely, when we eat less than our daily energy expenditure, we draw on our fat and carbohydrate stores to make up the deficit. We usually achieve energy balance over several days because of oscillations in over-eating and under-eating in relation to daily energy expenditure. A stable body weight for several days is a relatively good indicator of energy balance.

Energy intake = energy expenditure ± energy stored

Our daily energy expenditure is not a simple consequence of our physical activity but includes the energy expended to maintain all our bodily functions, including the cost of eating, digesting and absorbing our meals. The underpinning energy required to maintain all these physiological functions that support life is determined from measuring our metabolic rate while we are at complete rest. The basal metabolic rate (BMR) depends on our gender, age, height and weight and accounts for about 60% of our daily energy expenditure. An example of the distribution of daily energy expenditure of a 70 kg man is shown in Figure 22.3. In addition to BMR, there is the metabolic cost of physical activity (thermic effect of exercise, TEE) and the energy cost of digesting and absorbing our meals (thermic effect of feeding, TEF) which amounts to about 10% of our daily intake. In reality, resting metabolic (RMR) is measured because of the inconvenience of assessing of BMR in the morning,

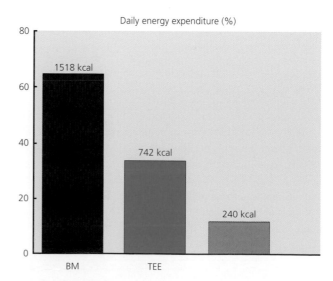

Figure 22.3 Energy intake and energy expenditure 70 kg man consuming 2500 kcal/day. TEE: thermic effect of exercise; TEF: thermic effect of feeding

Table 22.2 Harris benedict activity factors

Activity	Description	PAL factor
Low level	Largely sedentary, that is, little additional activity beyond that required for daily living	1.2
Mild level	Intensive exercise for at least 20 min about one to three times a week. Activities including jogging, cycling, swimming, football, hockey, rugby	1.375
Moderate level	Intensive exercise for at least 30–60 min a day for 3 to 4 days a week involving activities such as those listed above	1.55
Heavy level	Intensive exercise for 60 min or more for 5 to 7 days a week involving activities such as those listed above	1.7
Extreme level	Extremely active, for example, athletes involved in heavy training at least twice a day for most days of the week	1.9

shortly after waking. A good estimate of BMR can be calculated from the following formulae:

$$women\,(BMR) = 655 + (9.6 \times weight\,(kg)) + (1.8 \times height\,(cm))$$
$$-(4.7 \times age\,(year))$$
$$men\,(BMR) = 66 + (13.7 \times weight\,(kg)) + (5 \times height\,(cm))$$
$$-(6.8 \times age\,(year))$$

Knowing our BMR helps to estimate our total daily energy expenditure as follows:

$$energy\ expenditure = BMR \times physical\ activity\ level$$

Physical activity level (PAL) is less easily assessed because it requires a 'time and motion' analysis for all our daily activities. Nevertheless, using PAL, calculated from the Harris Benedict formula (Table 22.2), an estimate of the daily energy expenditure can be derived using multiples of BMR. It should be stressed that the level of activity is above and beyond that required for daily living. People who undertake very little physical activity are assigned a PAL of 1.2, whereas the value for athletes who train at least twice a day is 1.9. Professional cyclists on the 'Grand Tours' can sustain metabolic rates equivalent to 5 × BMR for most days of racing.

When body weight is constant, then the estimated daily energy expenditure reflects the energy intake of the individual. From these approximations of energy intake, the composition of daily food intake can be prescribed. Using the energy equivalents for carbohydrate (4 kcal g^{-1}), protein (4 kcal g^{-1}) and fat ((9 kcal g^{-1}), the energy intake of an individual can be translated into quantities of macronutrients in the diet. Using this information, the composition of a diet can be modified, for example, to increase the carbohydrate content without changing the overall energy intake.

Weight loss can only be achieved when we are in 'negative energy balance'. To lose 1 kg of body mass, we need to achieve a negative energy balance equivalent to about 7000 kcal. Decreasing food intake and increasing energy expenditure, even by small amounts is the most successful method of losing body weight. For example, reducing daily energy intake by 250 kcal for a month would bring about the desired body weight change of 1 kg. These approaches are

sustainable, and so an athlete could go onto lose a greater amount should it be required. One note of caution is that when body mass is reduced by 1 kg, about 25% is lean tissue.

Energy metabolism

The main fuels for energy production are carbohydrates and fat. Carbohydrate is stored as a glucose polymer (glycogen) in liver and skeletal muscle (see Figure 22.4): about 3 g of water is stored with every gram of glycogen. Liver glycogen provides glucose for brain metabolism, and it also supplements glycogen metabolism in skeletal muscles during exercise (see Figure 22.5). The average glycogen concentration is about 13 g kg^{-1} skeletal muscle, which makes up about 40% to overall body weight. Therefore, the glycogen content of skeletal muscle is about 360 g and yields approximately 4 kcal g^{-1} (16.7 kJ g^{-1}). Thus, the energy equivalent of skeletal muscle glycogen is about 1440 kcal (6019 kJ). In addition, the adult liver, weighing about 1.8 kg, contains approximatcly 90–100 g of glycogen and so, in total, the energy equivalent of stored carbohydrate is equivalent to about 2000 kcal.

Fat is stored in adipose tissue cells and in skeletal muscle as triglycerides. It is the main fuel during prolonged exercise. Complete oxidation of fat yields the equivalent of 9 kcal g^{-1} (37.6 kJ g^{-1}), and so the average 70 kg man (15% body fat) has approximately 94,500 kcal of energy stored as fat. Thus, the energy stored as carbohydrate is only 2% of the available energy stored as fat.

After a few minutes of submaximal exercise, oxygen demand is met by oxygen delivery and the resulting oxidation of fat and carbohydrate covers the energy (adenosine triphosphate, ATP) to support muscle contractions. However, the relative contributions are dependent on a number of physiological conditions. The first is the exercise intensity relative to the individual's maximum capacity for oxygen consumption (VO$_{2max}$). At low relative exercise intensities (<50% VO$_{2max}$), fat is the main fuel with only a minor contribution from carbohydrate metabolism. As exercise intensity increases, there is a greater contribution from carbohydrate metabolism: fatigue occurs when the stores of muscle glycogen are used up (micrograph 2). However, the carbohydrate used during exercise is not confined to muscle glycogen because blood glucose derived from the liver glycogen makes an ever increasing contributes to muscle metabolism during prolonged exercise.

During sprinting, the limiting influence on performance is the cellular decrease in muscle pH. Glycogenolysis makes a significant contribution to energy production during sprint, and as such there is an accumulation of hydrogen ions as a consequence of the production and dissociation of lactic acid. The capacity to perform repeated maximum sprints depends not only on delaying a severe reduction in muscle pH but also on the muscle's ability to rapidly resynthesise the small energy store of phosphocreatine (PCr) between sprints (see later).

Nutritional strategies

Before exercise

Recognising the central role carbohydrate plays in energy metabolism it is not surprising that nutritional strategies have

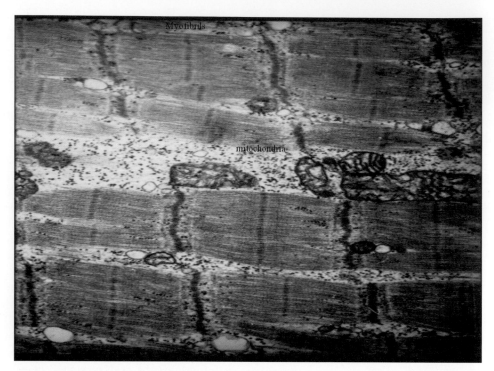

Figure 22.4 An electron photomicrograph of human skeletal muscle (inside one muscle fibre), which was obtained by percutaneous needle biopsy from the vastus lateralis muscle at rest before prolonged submaximal exercise to fatigue. The black dots between and within the myofibrils are glycogen granules: mitochondria are present between the myofibrils. Clear droplets of triglycerides are also visible although not as abundant as the glycogen granules

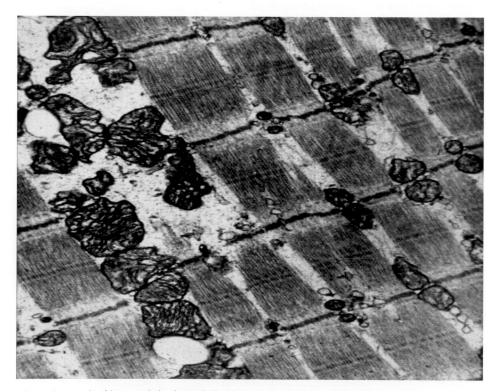

Figure 22.5 An electron photomicrograph of human skeletal muscle (inside one muscle fibre), which was obtained by percutaneous needle biopsy from the vastus lateralis muscle at the point of fatigue following prolonged submaximal exercise. The black dots between and within the myofibrils are glycogen granules: mitochondria are present between the myofibrils. Clear droplets of triglycerides are also visible although not as abundant as the glycogen granules

been developed to increase muscle glycogen stores before exercise. The most effective and acceptable method of carbohydrate loading is to decrease training 3–4 days before competition and increase the consumption of carbohydrate containing foods in each meal. Following very heavy training, then a carbohydrate intake of about 9–10 g kg^{-1} body weight is sufficient to replenish muscle and liver glycogen stores in preparation for another day of heavy training or competition. Eating an easy-to-digest high-carbohydrate meal 3–4 h before exercise helps top up glycogen stores mainly in the liver but not exclusively because there is some contribution to the muscle's store of glycogen.

During exercise

Dehydration causes fatigue during prolonged exercise even before the depletion of muscle glycogen. Drinking well-formulated carbohydrate–electrolyte solutions (sports drinks) throughout prolonged exercise helps prevent severe dehydration and contributes to carbohydrate metabolism in working muscles. Ingesting sports drinks that provide carbohydrate at a rate of about 60 g h^{-1} is effective in increasing endurance capacity. Athletes should relate their drinking to their rate of sweating, that is, when sweating heavily and then drink more than when sweat rates are low. Excess water intake will dilute the blood sodium concentration (hyponatremia) and cause a serious health risk. Therefore, it is safest to adopt the simple mantra 'drink a lot only when you sweat a lot'.

After exercise

Speed of recovery depends on how quickly muscle glycogen can be replaced and fluid balance restored. Glycogen resynthesis is most rapid during the first few hours after exercise. Therefore, consuming carbohydrate immediately after exercise takes advantage of the rapid period of glycogen resynthesis. Ingesting a sports drink is a convenient way of providing carbohydrate for glycogen synthesis as is eating HGI snacks. The optimum amount of carbohydrate is about 1 g kg^{-1} body weight, which is equivalent to about a litre of a sports drink containing 6% to 7% carbohydrate. In addition, consuming 50 g of carbohydrate every hour until the next meal is also an effective nutritional strategy to help achieve rapid glycogen repletion.

Protein synthesis is most rapid during recovery after resistance training when the ongoing dynamic balance between synthesis and degradation shifts towards greater synthesis. Post-exercise ingestion of foods that contain all the essential amino acids enhances protein synthesis in recovering skeletal muscles. Whey protein has all the essential amino acids that form the building blocks for new proteins. An excellent source of the essential amino acids is the whey protein in milk. Therefore, milk has been shown to be an effective post-exercise protein supplement because of its whey content.

Supplements

There are supplements galore with claims to have ergogenic benefits. Relatively few have acceptable research evidence to support their performance enhancing claims. Supplements that have an ergogenic benefits can be considered under four broad headings according to their function. They are (i) nutritional supplements that correct dietary deficiency/insufficiency; (ii) supplements that are concentrated foods providing easy access to additional fuel; (iii) supplements that are 'metabolic enhancers'; (iv) supplements that are stimulants that act on the central nervous system as well as on peripheral tissues.

Nutritional supplements

Sportspeople who under-eat (diet) in order to achieve or maintain a low fat mass are most at-risk of at least nutrient insufficiency and at worse nutrient deficiency. Iron-deficiency anaemia (Hb: <120 g l^{-1}) is relatively easy to detect, this is not the case with iron deficiency without anaemia. Therefore, assessment of iron deficiency (serum ferritin: <20.0 µg l^{-1}) should be included in the health checks on athletes with persistent fatigue. Supplementary iron provides nutritional 'first aid' until changes in diet are introduced to correct this deficiency.

Nitrates

Eating high nitrate containing foods such as spinach, lettuce and beetroot increase plasma nitrite via the nitric oxide (NO) synthase pathway. The increase in plasma nitric oxide has several beneficial effects on both the cardiovascular system and muscle metabolism. For example, (i) it reduces blood pressure, (ii) increases muscle blood flow, (iii) increases glucose uptake and (iv) improves efficiency of cellular energy production. For example, these changes reduce the oxygen cost of submaximal running and improve time trial performance during cycling, running and rowing. Consuming a concentrated beetroot juice for 5–6 days before exercise performance is the most frequently reported method of raising plasma nitrite concentrations.

Supplementary fuels
Creatine monohydrate

Creatine is one of the constituents of meat and fish: 1 g is equivalent to the creatine content of 1 kg of meat. Creatine is part of phosphocreatine (PCr) which is the body's 'starter fuel' (Figure 22.6).

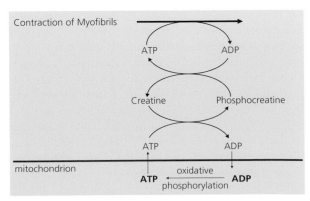

Figure 22.6 Creatine metabolisms. The mechanism by which creatine contributes to the resynthesis of phosphocreatine and thereafter the regeneration of ATP.

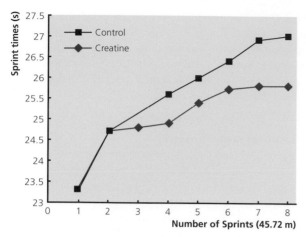

Figure 22.7 Influence of creatine supplementation (9 g per day for 5 days) on performance during sprint swimming (8 × 45.72 m, i.e. 50 yards) at intervals of 90 s (PB=personal best). Source: Adapted from Peyrebrune et al., 1988 "The effects of oral creatine supplementation on performance in single and repeated sprint swimming". Reproduced by permission of Taylor & Francis Ltd (http://www.informaworld.com)

For example, during the onset of exercise, there is a delay in the aerobic production of ATP and so the shortfall is largely covered by the degradation of phosphocreatine and glycogen. Power output during a series of maximum sprints with recovery of no more than 30 s between each sprint decreases because of an insufficient time for PCr resynthesis. Creatine supplementation increases its concentration as well as the PCr store in skeletal muscles. After supplementation, the decrease in power output during multiple sprints is less rapid than before supplementation. The effective dose of creatine monohydrate is 20–30 g per day for 5 to 6 days before exercise/competition. Creatine supplementation improves sprinting during running and cycling. However, low-dose supplementation also improves the performance of elite swimmers during interval training (Figure 22.7). It is important to note that body weight increases after several days of creatine supplementation because of an expansion of cellular water.

Metabolic-enhancing supplements
Bicarbonate loading
During brief periods of sprinting, glycogenolysis increases lactate and hydrogen ions concentrations that decrease cellular pH (Figure 22.8). The resulting acidity in muscle cells is associated with the onset of fatigue. Increasing the buffering capacity of the blood by the pre-exercise ingestion of a sodium bicarbonate solution increases the capacity to perform brief high-intensity exercise for short periods of time. The usual dose of bicarbonate is about 300 mg kg^{-1} body mass taken an hour or more before exercise. Higher doses cause gastrointestinal disturbances and, in some people, nausea and diarrhoea. The increased blood-buffering capacity encourages a rapid transfer of hydrogen ions out of the muscle cells and so helps restore intra-cellular pH more quickly to pre-exercise values. Pre-exercise bicarbonate loading improves performance times of middle distance runners and also the performance of elite swimmers during 50 m sprints.

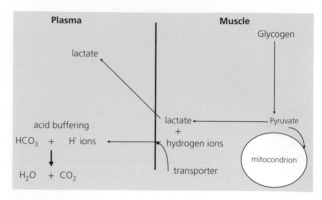

Figure 22.8 Bicarbonate metabolisms. The translocation of hydrogen ions out of muscle fibres.

Beta-alanine
As mentioned earlier, one of the limitations to sustained high-intensity exercise is the rapid formation of hydrogen ions that accompany the glycolytic surge to meet the high demands for ATP production. Within skeletal muscle, there are physiological buffers that help prevent an irreversible fall in cellular pH. Carnosine is one of the principal intra-cellular buffers and is found in greater amounts in fast-twitch muscle fibres. Fast-twitch fibres, recruited in large numbers during high-intensity exercise, generate ATP almost entirely by glycogenolysis with an accompanying rapid production of hydrogen ions. Beta-alanine contributes to the essential step in the production muscle carnosine. Four weeks of supplementation improves exercise capacity during brief high-intensity activities that last between 1 and 4 min. Earlier studies report that some participants experienced paraesthesia as a side effect of the supplementation, but this is not the case with a slow release beta-alanine.

Carnitine
An increase in fatty acid oxidation during exercise spares the limited muscle glycogen stores. Carnitine is a substrate for the enzyme carnitine palmitoyltransferase I, which is the rate-liming step in the transfer of fatty acids into mitochondria for oxidation. Recognising the central enabling role that carnitine plays in fat oxidation and then supplementing the diet with carnitine have long been suggested as a potential ergogenic aid. For example, supplementation with 2 g of L-carnitine along with 80 g of carbohydrate (to stimulate insulin release that facilitates carnitine translocation) twice daily for 24 weeks resulted in a 20% increase in muscle carnitine content and improved metabolic efficiency and exercise performance. During high-intensity exercise, the increased mitochondrial concentration of carnitine also helps achieve better matching of glycolytic, pyruvate dehydrogenase complex and mitochondrial flux leading to a reduction in anaerobic energy production and an increased work capacity.

Caffeine
Consuming caffeine in the form of strong coffee or in tablet form was used to increase the mobilisation of fatty acids from adipose

tissue cells. However, caffeine has a much more powerful effect on the central nervous system than on fat cells *per se*. It improves tolerance to high-intensity exercise, and even relatively small doses of caffeine have a significant ergogenic effect. Once thought to contribute to dehydration, this effect has been over-emphasised. Even no longer banned by the IOC, great care should be taken when using this ergogenic aid because 'more does not necessarily mean better' from a health and performance perspective.

Summary

Participants in sport and exercise should eat a well-balanced diet that contains a wide range of foods in order to cover their energy expenditure and maintain good health. As training load (intensity and duration) increases, athletes should consume more carbohydrate while attempting to maintain energy balance and so avoid gaining fat mass. Using commonly available foods in a strategic way will both support and enhance responses to training. Although there are ergogenic supplements that are effective in improving exercise performance, they tend to be specific to the type of exercise undertaken. However, there is no substitute for a well-structured individual training programme that is supported by a well-planned nutrition strategy.

Further reading

Burke, L.M., Hawley, J.A. & Wong, S.H. (2011) Carbohydrate for training and competition. *Journal of Sports Sciences*, **29** (**S1**), S17–S27.

Jeppesen, J. & Kiens, B. (2012) Regulation and limitations to fatty acid oxidation during exercise. *The Journal of Physiology*, **590** (**5**), 1059–1068.

Jeukendrup, A. & Gleeson, M. (2010) *Sport Nutrition*, 2nd edn. Human Kinetics, UK.

Loucks, A.B., Kiens, B. & Wright, H.H. (2011) Energy availability in athletes. *Journal of Sports Sciences*, **29** (**S1**), S7–S15.

Maughan, R.J., Greenhaff, P.L. & Hespel, P. (2011) Dietary supplements for athletes: emerging trends and recurring themes. *Journal of Sports Sciences*, **29** (**S1**), S57–S66.

Peyrebrune, M., Nevill, M., Donaldson, F. & Cosford, D. (1998) The effects of oral creatine supplementation on performance in single and repeated sprint swimming. *Journal of Sports Sciences*, **16** (**3**), 271–279.

Phillips, S.M. & Van Loon, L.J.C. (2011) Dietary protein for athletes: from requirements to optimum adaptation. *Journal of Sports Sciences*, **29** (**S1**), S29–S38.

CHAPTER 23

Drugs in Sport

Roger Palfreeman

Sport and Exercise Medicine, Claremont Hospital, Sheffield, UK

OVERVIEW

In this chapter we describe the area of drugs in sport. After studying this chapter, the reader will know

- The anti-doping agencies and their remit
- The substances prohibited at all times (in- and out-of competition)
- The methods prohibited at all times (in- and out-of competition)
- The substances and methods only prohibited in-competition
- The athlete biological passport (ABP)

Introduction

In the previous edition of this book, reference was made to a doping scandal involving the 1998 Tour de France cycle race, where a large number of doping products were discovered following a long period of undercover surveillance by the French Authorities.

In this edition, we are able to begin the chapter with, yet again, another major doping scandal. In 2013, Lance Armstrong, the seven-time winner of the Tour de France and one of the most successful sportsmen of all time, finally admitted to using performance enhancing drugs throughout his career. This had been the subject of considerable speculation for several years. However, the strongest evidence against him was not obtained from anti-doping tests, but from the witness statements of former colleagues provided to an investigation by United States Anti-Doping Agency (USADA). Armstrong had been subject to frequent testing procedures during his career and had never returned a positive result.

The World Anti-Doping Agency (WADA) was established in 1999. Its remit is to coordinate a worldwide response to doping by working with governments, public authorities and other involved bodies such as International Sports Federations, National Anti-Doping Organisations and the International Olympic Committee. WADA publishes a list of prohibited substances on an annual basis, which evolves to take account of new doping practices. In addition, there is a separate Monitoring Program,

ABC of Sports and Exercise Medicine, Fourth Edition.
Edited by Gregory P. Whyte, Mike Loosemore and Clyde Williams.
© 2015 John Wiley & Sons, Ltd. Published 2015 by John Wiley & Sons, Ltd.

whereby substances with potential for misuse are tested for when an athlete provides a sample. These results are not used to sanction an athlete, rather to inform WADA about emerging patterns of use of medications with potential for performance enhancement. Examples of substances on the Monitoring Program currently include in-competition use of Bupropion, nicotine and Tramadol and out-of-competition use of corticosteroids.

If an athlete has a medical requirement for any of the products on the prohibited list, they must first obtain a Therapeutic Use Exemption (TUE) certificate. This applies for many commonly used medicines, such as certain asthma inhalers, and corticosteroid use during or close to competition time. If a prohibited medicine is needed for emergency use, the medication can be given, then a retrospective application for a TUE can be made. The complete WADA list can be downloaded from their website (http://www.wada-ama.org/en/world-anti-doping-program/sports-and-anti-doping-organizations/international-standards/prohibited-list/), and the reader is strongly encouraged to obtain a copy of this document if they work in competitive sport.

Substances and methods prohibited at all times (in- and out-of-competition)

Prohibited substances
S0 Non-approved substances

This is a relatively new category that has been added to account for medications still under development or veterinary products that are not included in the other classifications.

S1 Anabolic agents
Anabolic androgenic steroids

This category includes a large number of steroid compounds, with notable inclusions being Nandrolone, Oxandrolone, Oxymetholone, Stanozolol and Methandienone. Low levels of Nandrolone are produced naturally in the body and, for this reason, threshold values of 2 and 5 ng ml^{-1} for males and females, respectively, have been set. Over the past few years, there have been a large number of positive tests with Nandrolone (19-Nortestosterone) metabolites above the permitted level, as well as those involving other anabolic steroids. Some athletes proclaim their innocence and attribute the findings to contaminated nutritional supplements, and studies have shown an alarmingly high prevalence of contamination in certain classes of supplements, particularly those offering gains in strength and muscle mass. In some instances, more potent steroids, such as Methanedieneone (Dianabol) and Stanozolol have also been discovered, raising the possibility that some manufacturers may be deliberately manipulating their products to cause greater effects on the user, thereby increasing sales.

Anabolic steroids

- Anabolic compounds are commonly found in nutritional supplements
- Meat from China and Mexico has been found to contain Clenbutarol
- The use of nutritional supplements should be monitored carefully and avoided wherever possible

---

The situation regarding contamination has been compounded by improved detection methods for many anabolic steroids, with approval for the use of long-term metabolites (LTMs) as a marker of abuse. These are metabolites of the original steroid that persist long after the original drug is no longer detectable.

Tetrahydrogestrinone (THG) was one of the first 'designer steroids'. This term is reserved for steroids with no known therapeutic indication, whose structure has been modified to make it difficult to detect by anti doping laboratories. It is structurally similar to Gestrinone, which is used to treat endometriosis. In 2003, the existence of this new steroid was brought to the attention of USADA, who subsequently arranged for the retesting of a number of urine samples from prominent athletes and found evidence of THG use in several cases (the BALCO scandal). In the following 5-year period, 22 such 'designer steroids' with no known therapeutic use were identified, and more have emerged since then.

Other anabolic agents
This category includes Clenbutarol and Zeranol. Both have been used as growth promoters in the beef industry. Zeranol is a non-steroidal oestrogen analogue, which is only for veterinary use. Clenbutarol is a beta-2 agonist, also used in the treatment of asthma in humans in some EC countries, but not in the United Kingdom. There is some evidence from animal studies that Clenbutarol can produce anabolic effects on muscle and reduce adipose tissue via beta-2 receptor action. Of concern is the fact that meat, particularly from certain countries such as China and Mexico, may be contaminated by Clenbutarol and inadvertently ingested by athletes. It is now accepted that this has been responsible for several adverse analytical findings (AAFs) over the past 2–3 years. Furthermore, Clenbutarol has also been found as an unlisted constituent in nutritional products promoted as 'fat burners'.

Selective Androgen Receptor Modulators (SARMs) are included in this category. These are non-steroid compounds that act on androgen receptors in muscle and bone, with reduced effects on other tissues. While there are currently no SARMs with a license as a therapeutic medication, Ostarine is currently in phase 3 clinical trials and a number of these experimental drugs have been abused by athletes.

S2 Peptide hormones, growth factors and related compounds
This category contains many of the products known to be widely abused in a variety of different sports.

(i) Erythropoiesis-stimulating agents (ESAs), for example, erythopoietin, darbepoietin, hypoxia-inducible factor (HIF) stabilisers, continuous erythropoietin receptor activator (CERA), peginesatide (hematide)
(ii) Human chorionic gonadotrophin (hCG), luteinising hormone (LH) and their releasing factors (prohibited in males only)
(iii) Corticotrophins
(iv) Human growth hormone (hGH) and insulin-like growth factor (IGF-1)

In addition, certain growth factors, including those acting on muscle, tendon and blood vessels, are prohibited.

Erythropoiesis stimulating agents
Erythropoietin (EPO) is a glycoprotein hormone produced by the kidney. It acts on erythroid precursors in the bone marrow to increase the rate of red blood cell production, thereby improving the ability of the blood to transport oxygen. In the late 1980s, recombinant (synthetic) EPO became available and its use by professional road cyclists and cross-country skiers, in particular, became widespread. By the mid-to-late 1990s, there was evidence that some professional cyclists were riding with a haematocrit of up to 65%, similar to residents living at extreme high altitudes! Furthermore, this was often accompanied by intravenous iron infusions in the belief that oral iron supplementation was not adequate to support such accelerated rates of erythrocyte formation. Iron overload became common, with ferritin levels often in excess of $1000 \, \text{ng ml}^{-1}$, similar to the levels that occur in hereditary haemochromatosis.

Since then, a number of modified forms of EPO have become available, as well as structurally unrelated compounds that are also capable of acting on the EPO receptor and stimulating erythropoiesis. New drugs are under investigation, and some of these (HIF stabilisers) target the hypoxia-sensing mechanism in the kidneys rather than the EPO receptor itself. Furthermore, in 2004, the European patent for recombinant EPO expired and this allowed for the manufacturing of 'biosimilar products'. These are EPO copy products that do not have to undergo clinical trials or any form of testing procedure prior to their use. They are structurally similar, but not identical to the original product and, in some cases, the modification can make them very difficult to detect by conventional anti-doping tests. At least 80 biosimilars are currently available.

Detection of ESA abuse currently involves the use of two complementary methods, *direct* and *indirect*. The direct method relies on the detection of the actual ESA itself (most often EPO) from molecular fragments in a urine sample. Unfortunately, this test, pioneered in the French National Anti-Doping Laboratory, has relatively low sensitivity. Sensitivity is further reduced if the drug is taken in a regime known as 'microdosing'. In microdosing, the athlete takes low doses daily, as opposed to therapeutic doses taken less frequently. Furthermore, administration of the drug via the intravenous route results in a shorter half-life than the subcutaneous route. This makes detection of the banned product more difficult.

Long-acting forms of rhEPO, such as darbepoietin and CERA, have become available since the advent of EPO therapy. These allow patients (and unscrupulous athletes) to reduce the frequency of administration. However, the long half-life and molecular modification make their detection as a doping agent relatively easy by the direct method.

A major breakthrough in the fight against doping has been the introduction of a new *indirect* approach to the detection of banned substances – the athlete biological passport (ABP) – which seeks to detect not the actual drug itself, but the effects of the product on the body. The ABP lends itself very well to the problem of blood doping, where the continual development of new ESAs and biosimilars has made direct detection problematic. In addition, the administration of blood transfusions can also be revealed in this way. Most recently, steroid profiling has been added to the ABP system and, in future, it is likely that other prohibited substances and methods will also be included. The Biological Passport will be discussed in more detail in a later section of this chapter.

ESAs

- Are widely abused in endurance sports
- Are still difficult to detect, despite tests being available
- The ABP is a new method of identifying ESA use
- Many EPO biosimilars now exist in addition to the original forms

---

Corticotrophins

Tetracosactrin (Synacthen) consists of the first 24 N-terminal amino acids of adrenocorticotrophic hormone (ACTH). It is given by injection and acts on the adrenal cortex to promote the secretion of glucocorticosteroids. The plasma half-life of Tetracosactrin is in the order of a few minutes, making detection extremely difficult. It is used primarily in endurance sports instead of or as an adjunct to systemic corticosteroids, and its effects are likely to be similar to those discussed previously.

Growth hormone (rhGH) and insulin-like growth factor (IGF-1)

These two related products are thought to be abused by both strength and endurance athletes. There is a general belief that they are effective in building muscle and reducing adipose tissue. There is very little evidence in the literature, however, to support a performance enhancing effect for either drug when used in isolation. In practice, they are commonly used along with insulin or anabolic steroids, so their true effect remains unknown. What is beyond doubt is their potential for adverse effects, including permanent skeletal changes and cardiomyopathy. Furthermore, since most rhGH is obtained on the black market, there is no guarantee that the product supplied contains any active hormone. In some cases, inactive bovine GH or human chorionic gonadotrophin are substituted. There are now two different methods for detecting GH abuse, and the first positive finding was obtained in 2010, following which several other athletes have returned positive doping test results. However, there is still no method of detecting IGF-1 abuse.

Growth hormone

- Used by strength and endurance athletes
- There is only weak evidence of performance enhancement
- Potential for severe side effects
- Detection methods are now available

S3 Beta-2 agonists

Salbutamol (maximum dose 1600 µg per 24 h), Formoterol (54 µg per 24 h) and Salmeterol are permitted by inhalation only to prevent/treat asthma and exercise-induced bronchoconstriction. Other beta-2 agonists, such as Terbutaline, require a TUE. However, if the urinary concentration of Salbutamol exceeds 1000 ng ml^{-1} or the level of Formoterol is greater than 40 ng ml^{-1}, it will be considered an AAF unless the athlete is able to prove, through a pharmacokinetic study, that the abnormal result is a consequence of therapeutic use that does not exceed the maximum stipulated doses.

Beta-2 agonists

- Are permitted by inhalation only
- Salbutamol levels >1000 ng ml^{-1} are considered an AAF, irrespective of a TUE

S4 Hormone and metabolic modulators

This category contains a number of different classes of compound, including aromatase inhibitors, and other oestrogenic substances, which are principally used to reduce the oestrogenic side effects of anabolic steroid use in males, such as gynaecomastia.

A recent addition to S4 are myostatin inhibitors and related substances, capable of modifying the action of the myostatin gene within skeletal muscle. Myostatin normally functions to prevent excessive skeletal muscle growth, and inhibition of its function might therefore be expected to lead to muscle hypertrophy. A number of myostatin inhibitors are currently in clinical trials to assess their therapeutic use in a variety of muscle wasting disorders and they have obvious potential for abuse by athletes.

Several experimental drugs thought to act on the intracellular signalling pathways in skeletal muscle are found in the S4 category. GW1516 is an agonist of the Peroxisome Proliferator Activated Receptor (PPAR-delta) complex, while AICAR acts on the amputee (AMP)-activated protein kinase axis. There is evidence that both are able to mimic the effects of endurance training on muscle via the upregulation of specific genes, resulting in improved performance. There are reports that both have been used by endurance athletes.

Insulin may be ergogenic via its inhibition of protein degradation and probably acts synergistically with GH to generate an anabolic effect. In addition, it promotes muscle glycogen synthesis secondary to increased glucose uptake, which may help to explain why it is used by endurance athletes such as professional road cyclists when competing in stage races. Use of insulin is only permitted by diabetics, who must first obtain a TUE.

S5 Diuretics and other masking agents

A number of chemically unrelated substances are used to hide the presence of a banned substance. Examples include plasma expanders such as hydroxyethyl starch or human albumin solution. These can transiently lower the haemoglobin concentration in those who have been using ESAs or blood transfusions.

Diuretics are used to dilute the urine sample and promote excretion of banned substances, reducing the chance of detection.

Prohibited methods

M1 Manipulation of blood and blood components

Blood transfusion

Can be autologous (own blood) or homologous (cross-matched blood taken from a donor). In autologous transfusion, blood is taken from the circulation and then re-infused after a delay of several weeks (during which time the bone marrow replenishes the blood that has been removed). Blood transfusion had become largely redundant following the development of rhEPO. However, with the advent of tests capable of detecting rhEPO use, these practices have re-emerged. Homologous transfusion involves erythrocytes that are cross-matched for ABO and Rhesus (D) compatibility, but not usually for minor blood group antigens. Such 'foreign' antigens can now be identified at least 4 weeks after administration, making this method of blood doping relatively easy to detect. Unfortunately, there is still no definitive (direct) method for detecting autologous transfusions, but specific patterns in the haematological profile of the Biological Passport can be strongly suggestive of this form of doping.

Blood transfusion

- Can be autologous (own blood) or homologous (donor blood)
- Homologous transfusions are easily detected
- Autologous transfusions are more difficult to detect but their use may be apparent on the Biological Passport

---

Products that enhance the uptake, transport or delivery of oxygen include haemoglobin-based oxygen carriers (HBOCs). These contain non-cellular haemoglobin of bovine, human or recombinant origin. The most advanced product is Hemopure, which is licensed in South Africa for treatment of acute blood loss. Despite the potential for abuse in sport and some earlier anecdotal reports of its use, any performance enhancing effects may be lost at workloads approaching VO_{2max} due to its potent vasoconstrictor effect. Recent use of Hemopure can now be detected in a blood sample.

Other products included in the M1 category include perfluorocarbons (synthetic emulsions that readily dissolve oxygen) and allosteric haemoglobin effectors, which act by stabilising the deoxygenated form of haemoglobin, thereby facilitating the offloading of oxygen.

M2 Chemical and physical manipulation

This refers to the use of methods or substances that alter the integrity of the urine/blood sample. It includes urine substitution, reducing renal excretion of proscribed drugs and altering testosterone/epitestosterone ratios. Of particular note is the recent inclusion of proteases; enzymes capable of degrading the urinary peptide fragments of EPO, thereby confounding the direct urine test for this drug. Proteases were added to the prohibited list when it became apparent that athletes were introducing them into the urine sample provided at doping control by first contaminating their fingers with protease-containing substances, such as biological washing powder, then allowing some urine to pass over them while providing a specimen!

M3 Gene doping

It is already possible to introduce the EPO gene into non-EPO producing cells in other primates. When this was performed on baboons, however, the haematocrit rose rapidly from 40% to 75% in the space of 10 weeks and regular venesection was then required to prevent death. Similar experiments have been carried out using the GH gene. The main limitation to the use of such technology in humans is the subsequent lack of control over hormone production. Once this barrier has been removed, we might expect to see such methods used in sport. The WADA is currently supporting research to develop methods to detect gene doping.

Substances and methods prohibited in-competition only

S6 Stimulants

Examples include amphetamine and methylamphetamine as well as substances commonly found in over-the-counter (OTC) cold remedies, such as ephedrine and methylephedrine. For the majority of these products, the mere presence of the compound in the urine sample denotes a positive test. In the case of ephedrine and methylephedrine, there is a threshold limit of $10\,\mu g\,ml^{-1}$. Pseudoephedrine has a threshold limit of $150\,\mu g\,ml^{-1}$. There have been several recent cases where the presence of Methylhexaneamine (MHA) was attributed to the use of a sports nutrition supplement (with the MHA listed on the ingredients). Oxilofrine has been found as an unlisted contaminant in such products and has been responsible for a number of positive findings.

Stimulants

- Mild stimulants are commonly found in OTC medicines
- They can also be found in sport nutrition supplements, either listed or unlisted in the ingredients
- All such products should be thoroughly checked before use by competitive sports people
- Caffeine is not banned
- Pseudoephedrine is prohibited if the urinary concentration exceeds $150\,\mu g\,ml^{-1}$

Caffeine, phenylephrine, pseudoephedrine (below $150\,\mu g\,ml^{-1}$) and several other mild stimulants are included as part of the Monitoring Program. WADA will continue to test for these substances in order to detect any pattern of misuse. If evidence of abuse emerges, such as very high urinary concentrations, WADA reserves the right to replace them on the proscribed list. This reflects the fact that many of the positive tests for stimulants have come from inadvertent administration in OTC medicines taken to relieve minor ailments.

S7 Narcotics

Examples of these include all potent opioids, such as morphine, pethidine and diamorphine. Dihydrocodeine, codeine, pholcodine and other weak opioids are permitted. These are proscribed due to their potential for dependence and harm to the athlete, rather than any ergogenic effect. They can also be used to mask the pain of injuries with the attendant risk of further damage.

Tramadol is an atypical opioid, with additional serotonergic and noradrenergic properties, and is strongly suspected of being widely abused in certain sports, where its analgesic properties are thought to allow the athlete to perform at a higher level as a result of improved pain tolerance. There are anecdotal reports of professional road cyclists taking tramadol in amounts several times greater than the maximum therapeutic dose. It is thought that this may, in certain cases, have contributed to the rider crashing, quite possibly due to the drug's side effects, which include dizziness and drowsiness. It is currently on the Monitoring Program.

S8 Cannabinoids

Cannabinoids (e.g. Cannabis) are prohibited, once again, due to their potential to cause harm rather than gain any sporting advantage.

S9 Glucocorticosteroids

Corticosteroids are banned during competition when administered by the oral, intravenous, intramuscular or rectal routes. All other forms of administrations such as nasal sprays, inhalers, creams and soft tissue injections are permitted at all times. There is usually no restriction on corticosteroid use out of competition except in certain sports, where injections of any type are prohibited for a period of time prior to, and including, any competition. In the case of cycling, this exclusion period is for 8 days before competition.

Systemic corticosteroids are widely abused in some endurance sports, where they are used for a number of reasons. Anecdotally, they are thought to result in the breakdown of adipose tissue, particularly when combined with high volumes of endurance training. This effect is used primarily in endurance sports where the power-to-weight ratio is an important determinant of performance. While direct evidence of this effect is lacking, corticosteroids are known to dramatically elevate the levels of free fatty acids (FFA) in the blood. There are several studies that show elevated FFA are capable of causing mitochondrial uncoupling in muscle, resulting in reduced efficiency of contraction and increased energy expenditure. This probably only applies to low-intensity exercise, where FFA are the predominant fuel, so that muscular efficiency approaches normal as the workload increases. The raised levels of FFA also promote the use of lipids as fuel during exercise, resulting in sparing of muscle and liver glycogen. In addition, high doses may potentiate the effects of catecholamines on the cardiovascular system, thereby producing a secondary sympathomimetic effect.

The main mechanism of action of corticosteroids, however, may well involve a reduced perception of pain via a central effect, leading to significantly improved performance in sustained exercise. It's likely that several days of high-dose administration are needed for this to occur.

The long-term consequences of corticosteroid use can be significant. Adrenal suppression can occur, and this could results in a medical emergency when an athlete is acutely unwell or involved in trauma. There are also potential adverse effects on the cardiovascular system and on bone, as well as a number of other medical complications.

The athlete biological passport (ABP)

The ABP was introduced in 2009 as an alternative approach to the detection of doping. Rather than rely on the identification of a specific doping agent in a blood or urine sample, the ABP uses a panel of biomarkers to indirectly reveal the effects of doping on the body. This has a particular advantage in relation to blood doping, where new drugs capable of stimulating red blood cell formation are being continually developed, such that direct analytical methods fail to keep pace with doping practices. There are currently two modules in the ABP, the original haematology module and the steroid module, which appeared in 2014.

The basic principle with both modules is the same. Over a period of time, blood and urine samples are collected on an individual athlete to form their own Biological Passport. As more results are added to the passport, the software gradually learns what is typical for that athlete and individual reference ranges for each biomarker are established. In this way, the ABP is able to detect statistically unusual sequences of samples that might indicate doping, as well as single suspicious values.

The haematology biomarkers include haemoglobin concentration and reticulocytes. A high-haemoglobin concentration with low reticulocytes would be suggestive of a blood transfusion or recent cessation of ESA use, while low haemoglobin and high reticulocytes would be compatible with blood withdrawal (for subsequent transfusion) or commencement of ESA use. Changes in reticulocytes are seen as particularly significant and, for this reason, there are very strict quality controls over the collection of blood, its transportation and laboratory analysis of all samples. However, such changes as described can, on occasions, also be physiological or due to medical conditions. When a suspicious profile is seen, it is first sent out for review by a panel of experts. If the consensus is that the profile may be indicative of doping, the athlete is given the opportunity to offer an explanation for the anomalies. If this does not clarify the situation, a decision may be made to issue a passport violation, which is essentially a positive doping test. On other occasions, the expert recommendation may be to monitor the athlete more closely with targeted ABP testing, as well as random direct tests in order to find proof of EPO use, for example.

While the indirect ABP approach has great merit, there is evidence that it has resulted in changes in doping practices in an attempt to normalise the haematological profile. Use of a microdosing regime, where small doses of an ESA are used daily, or microtransfusions, where reduced volumes of blood are transfused every few days, are still difficult to detect, even with the ABP. Despite this, there appears to have been a significant reduction in abnormal haematological values since it was first introduced, suggesting the ABP is having a marked deterrent effect.

The recently introduced steroid module involves the measurement of testosterone and some of its metabolites in a urine sample. Over time, a steroid profile is built up, in much the same way as the blood profile. If any suspicious values or sequences emerge, the samples will be further evaluated with a more complex and involved analytical method known as Isotope Ratio Mass Spectrometry (IRMS). Only if the IRMS is negative, then the profile will be reviewed by a panel of experts and a decision be made on whether to issue a passport violation.

It is likely that the ABP adaptive model with be further expanded to include an endocrine module in the near future.

Summary box

1 All those working or competing in competitive sport should make themselves familiar with the WADA prohibited list.
2 Some common OTC medicines contain proscribed substances.
3 A number of nutritional supplements have been shown to be contaminated by anabolic substances and stimulants.
4 Competitive sportspeople should keep their use of such supplements to an absolute minimum to avoid the possibility of an inadvertent positive dope test.
5 The detection of banned substances and methods is improving, and the introduction of the ABP is a major step forward in the fight against doping in sport.

Further reading

Ashenden, M., Gough, C.E., Garnham, A., Gore, C.J. & Sharpe, K. (2011) Current markers of the Athlete Blood Passport do not flag microdose EPO doping. *European Journal of Applied Physiology*, 111, 2307–2314.

Duclos, M. (2010) Evidence on ergogenic action of glucocorticoids as a doping agent risk. *Physician and Sportsmed*, 3 (38), 121–127.

Gaudard, A., Varlet-Marie, E., Berssolle, F. & Audran, M. (2003) Drugs for increasing oxygen transport and their potential use in doping. *Sports Medicine.*, 33 (3), 187–212.

Geyer, H., Bredehoft, M., Marek, U., Parr, M.K. & Schanzer, W. (2003) High doses of the anabolic steroid Metandienone found in dietary supplements. *The European Journal of Sports Science*, 3 (1), 1–5.

Geyer, H., Schaenzer, W. & Thevis, M. (2014) Anabolic agents: recent strategies for their detection and protection from inadvertent doping. *British Journal of Sports Medicine*, 48 (10), 820–119.

Grond, S. & Sablotzki, A. (2004) Clinical pharmacology of tramadol. *Clinical Pharmacokinetics*, 43 (13), 879–923.

Guha, N., Cowan, D. & Soenksen, P. (2013) Insulin-like growth factor-I (IGF-I) misuse in athletes and potential methods for detection. *Analytical and Bioanalytical Chemistry*, 405, 9669–9683.

Leigh-Smith, S. (2004) Blood boosting. *British Journal of Sports Medicine*, 38, 99–101.

Macdougall, C. (2008) Novel erythropoiesis-stimulating agents: a new era in anemia management. *Clinical Journal of the American Society of Nephrology*, 3, 200–207.

Morkeberg, J. (2013) Blood manipulation: current challenges from an anti-doping perspective. *Hematology – American Society of Hematology Education Programs*, 2013, 627–631.

Mottram, D.R. (ed) (2010) *Drugs in Sport*. Taylor & Francis, Abingdon, Oxon.

Narkar, V.A. *et al.* (2008) AMPK and PPARδ agonists are exercise mimetics. *Cell*, 134 (3), 405–415.

Nelson, M., Popp, H., Sharpe, K. & Ashenden, M. (2003) Proof of homologous blood transfusion through quantification of blood group antigens. *Haematologica*, 88 (1), 1284–1295.

Peltre G, and Thorman W. (2003). *Evaluation report of the EPO blood tests.* WADA report

Pitsiladis, Y., Durusse, J. & Rabin, O. (2014) An integrative 'Omics' solution to the detection of recombinant human erythropoietin and blood doping. *British Journal of Sports Medicine*, 48, 856–861.

Pottgiesser, T., Sottas, P.E., Echteler, T., Robinson, N., Umhau, M. & Schumacher, Y.O. (2011) Detection of autologous blood doping with adaptively evaluated biomarkers of doping: a longitudinal blinded study. *Transfusion*, 51, 1707–1715.

Rennie, M.J. (2003) Claims for the anabolic effects of growth hormone: a case of the Emperor's new clothes? *British Journal of Sports Medicine*, 37, 100–105.

Saugy, M., Lundby, C. & Robinson, N. (2014) Monitoring of biological markers indicative of doping: the athlete biological passport. *British Journal of Sports Medicine*, 48, 827–883.

Schanzer, W (2002). *Analysis of non-hormonal nutritional supplements for androgenic anabolic steroids.* IOC report.

Schumacher, Y.O., Schmid, A., Dinkelmann, S., Berg, A. & Northoff, H. (2001) Artificial oxygen carriers – the new doping threat in endurance sport? *International Journal of Sports Medicine*, 22, 566–571.

Smith, R.C. & Lin, B.K. (2013) Myostatin inhibitors as therapies for muscle wasting associated with cancer and other disorders. *Current Opinion in Supportive and Palliative Care*, 7 (4), 352–360.

WADA (2003) *Independent observer report – Tour de France* 2003

CHAPTER 24

Psychology of Injury

Andrew M. Lane

Institute of Sport, Faculty of Education, Health and Well-being, University of Wolverhampton, Wolverhampton, UK

OVERVIEW

In this chapter we describe the psychology of injury. After studying this chapter, the reader will know

- Examination of how an athlete's psychological state could influence the rehabilitation process
- Description of how emotions unfold during injury
- Examination of how a physician's treatment could influence the psychological state of the injured athlete
- The role of goals and emotions in the rehabilitation process
- Description of practical strategies a physician could use to help an athlete recover psychologically with a particular focus on emotion management

Although participating in sport, exercise and physical activity has numerous physical and psychological benefits, incurring an injury is a common occurrence. As people exercise into old age, having effective coping strategies becomes even more important. Injuries can happen after or during a period of hard training when the athlete is aware of the stresses and strains being placed on their structures; at other times, injuries occur suddenly and unexpectedly. The consequence of both types of injuries is a reduction or cessation of training. This leads to a revision of athletic goals, and an intense emotional response. Many athletes tie a great deal of their self-esteem into the achievement of athletic goals, uncertainty on whether, or if, the athlete will be able to keep striving to achieve these goals influences emotions. The psychological effects of this process can be deep-rooted affecting thoughts and emotions and characterised by feeling downhearted, frustrated and angry. These intense emotional responses occur outside of the main issue being treated. The role of the doctor is to focus on treatment on physical effects of the injury. While psychological factors are appreciated, rarely are they the focus of specific treatment. The aim of this chapter is to describe how a physician's treatment may affect psychological recovery of the athlete. In addition, some consideration will be given to how treatment may affect the athlete's recovery

goals as well as the emotions and motivation that collectively could influence adherence to a rehabilitation programme.

Two issues that influence the recovery process will be covered. First is the influence of the feedback from the doctor (physician) on an athlete's goals and emotions Second, some practical strategies that the doctor could use to manage expectations will be covered regarding the speed of the recovery process and the client's mood. The guiding message is that the doctors could consider emotion management a part of the treatment plan.

How does injury affect goals and emotions?

When the medical team first treats an athlete suspected of suffering from a major injury, it is likely that the athlete will be struggling to come to terms with the effect of the injury. Injury is a negative outcome and one that signals uncertainty about the potential for achieving both short and long-term goals. The athlete is likely to experience intense emotions. Unpleasant emotions such as anger and depression signal that all is not well in the athlete's world while pleasant emotions such as happiness and excitement signal all is well or going well. Emotions can affect the success of the rehabilitation process, particularly through their influence on thoughts and behaviour. For example, if an individual misses a rehabilitation session, then unpleasant thoughts and feelings that stem from this might prompt him/her to promise to follow the programme more closely in the future. In this instance, the message learned was that if you want to avoid experiencing this unpleasant state in the future, then stick to the plan. However, emotions can be dysfunctional to goal achievement. Extending the above example, missing a session might lead to sadness and guilt, and the individual might learn that the best way to avoid experiencing these emotions is to abandon the goal in the first place and dropping out from the sport is considered. In both examples, emotion carried an important message, and this message influenced thoughts and action.

Researchers have proposed that there is a process that people go through when injured (see Figure 24.1). It should be noted that this was developed for people going through the grief process and then applied to sports injury. It is important to note that people can go through this process at different rates. People can interpret and appraise each process differently. It is also possible for someone to get stuck in one stage of the process, particularly the

---

ABC of Sports and Exercise Medicine, Fourth Edition.
Edited by Gregory P. Whyte, Mike Loosemore and Clyde Williams.

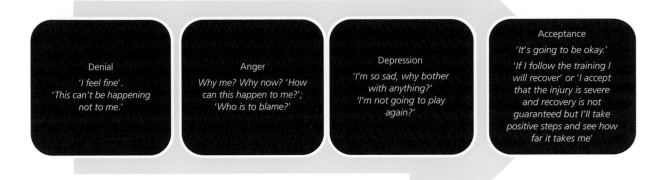

Figure 24.1 The Kublar–Ross model applied to sports injury

denial stage, and believe the injury is not as severe as the diagnosis. As a consequence, they are not likely to engage in rehabilitation exercisers and possibly believe that a few days rest will suffice. The aim is to accelerate the person through the process to the point the athlete accepts the injury; once accepted it is possible to establish realistic goals for recovery and identify the work required to deliver these goals.

How the doctor can influence emotion?

It is important that the doctor is aware that he/she can influence the goals and emotions of the athlete. The athlete places a great deal of importance on getting back to training and the doctor holds information and knowledge that can help that process. The athlete has expectations on how severe the injury is and what he/she needs to do to resume training. When the doctor provides feedback that indicates recovery is slow or slower than the athlete's expectations, this feedback could lead to an increase in unpleasant emotions. Feedback that indicates recovery is faster than expected leads to pleasant emotions.

How mood might influence the presentation of an injury

When treating an athlete the doctor should bear in mind that the athlete's emotions could influence how the athlete presents her/himself. If the athlete is feeling depressed by the injury, this could result in her or him presenting the injury as more severe than if he/she was happy. Although this is not routine practice, assessing an athlete's psychological state at the time of presentation of the injury through completion of a brief mood state scale (see Box 24.1)

Box 24.1 A typical mood measure

Mood is assessed using self-report measures where people look at words that describe their feeling and then assign a rating which indicates the intensity in which they are feeling this mood. For example, in the Brunel Mood Scale, the instructions to participants are:

Below is a list of words that help you describe how you are feeling today. Please read each one carefully. **Then circle the answer that best describes how you feel right now.** *Make sure you respond to every word.*

	Not at all	A little	Moderately	Quite a bit	Extremely
1. Angry	0	1	2	③	4
2. Confused	0	1	2	3	④
3. Depressed	0	1	2	③	4
4. Energetic	0	①	2	3	4
5. Nervous	0	1	②	3	4
6. Worn-out	0	1	2	③	4

is one approach. The simple guiding message is that unpleasant information (anger, confusion, depression, fatigue and tension) could associate something is wrong in the athletes environment and this might lead to presenting the information with greater severity than if the athlete was in a pleasant mood (see Figure 24.2). Monitoring mood throughout the injury process (recovery & rehabilitation) has been found to be a useful way of gaining inroads into the extent to which the athlete is making positive adaptations. The doctor should also be mindful of the influence of her/his actions on the emotional state of the athlete. At the point of consultation, the athlete is looking for reassurance that all is well or for some

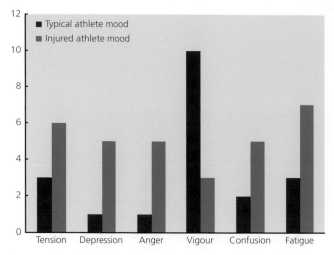

Figure 24.2 Mood state of a normal athlete (using normative data) and an injured athlete using the Brunel Mood Scale

Table 24.1 Guidelines for the goal-setting process

Goal setting	Description
Specific	Goals work by helping you to mobilise the amount of effort needed. To do that you need to know what you need to do. Example: 'My first goal is to do 10 reps at this 5 kg and do 3 sets in the rehabilitation session'.
	Typical issue: people set vague goals where they are not clear on whether it was achieved or not. For example, I will be good at doing my rehabilitation sessions – the individual will not know what counts as a good session.
Measureable	Goals should be measurable so that you need to know you have achieved it. The goal above was measureable due to the fact that the number of set and the weight were specified.
Attainable	The goal should be challenging, possibly very difficult, but it also should be attainable. An excessively difficult will demotivate. When someone is injured their capabilities are effected and this influences what they can do. People often try to get back too early and become despondent at failure. It is important to work on the notion that training should be progressive and achieving goals builds confidence.
Regularly reviewed	Progress toward the goal should be reviewed and checked regularly.
Timed	A timeline for goals allows you to establish the process by which to achieve them.

indication on the time-course of the recovery so that he/she can return to training and competition

A doctor should consider the how feedback influences the psychological state of the athlete. Injury should be seen as a continuum from its onset to recovery and return to training, however it is important to recognise how they rate of recovery may affect the emotions of athletes. People monitor the rate of progress toward achieving their goal. It has been argued that all behaviour is directed toward achieving a goal. A goal could be something grandiose such as winning an Olympic medal, or it could be something far less impressive like achieving under 4 h in a marathon. For example, if someone is sitting down and wants to stand up, the goal for that action is the capability to stand. Whilst this goal seems highly achievable most of the time, when an athlete is injured this can the type of goal that someone is working toward. Injury can affect confidence to do many day-to-day tasks that are done normally with confidence.

If the rate of progress towards the goal is faster or slower than the standard required, there will be a concomitant change in emotions. If the person wants to stand up, but has trouble doing so, which is reasonable during an injury, then the emotions such as frustration are likely to increase in intensity. If the person wants to stand up and does so effortlessly, then no change in emotion is likely. An injured athlete could be the former example and experiencing difficulty doing simple day-to-day challenges could influence emotions. The combined effect of finding simple tasks difficult to deal with can lead to unpleasant emotions accompanied by thoughts that signal low self-confidence to achieve even the most mundane tasks. In short, the injured person begins to adopt a state of learned-helplessness, a state where they rely almost entirely on the support of others. If athletes develop a state of learned helplessness, then the route to recovery is likely to be slower than expected because successful rehabilitation requires a great amount of personal motivation. For these reasons, it is important to help athlete's set goals that raise motivation (see Table 24.1).

If an individual recognises that the emotion experienced is not helpful in achieving defined goals then goals may be modified or

Box 24.2 Using music to help you change your mood

- Pay attention to the tempo of music when setting up folders to relax or energise; fast tempi are associated with higher arousal levels than slow tempi.
- Match the tempo of music with the intensity of exercise. For example, when cycling at around 70% of aerobic capacity, mid-tempo music (115–125 beats per minute) is more effective than faster music (135–145 beats per minute).
- Select music where the lyrics have a great deal of meaning.
- Select music that matches the task; for example with repetitive sports such as cycling, running and rowing, synchronise music to the movements. This can work for rehabilitation exercises also. If what you are doing is continuous then music could help.
- Encourage athletes to visualise themselves performing when listening to music.
- Encourage athletes to choose music that suits their taste and cultural upbringing.
- Reflect on the efficacy of song selection and update regularly.

an emotion regulation strategy adopted. There are 100 of different types of emotion regulation strategies including behavioural strategies such as exercise, listening to music, talking to someone, drinking alcohol, eating, etc. Listening to music is a particularly effective strategy as the choice of music can be selected in relation to the activity and mood required (Box 24.2).

There are also cognitive strategies (Table 24.2) such as re-appraising the task so that the athlete perceives it as attainable

Table 24.2 Changing unwanted emotions thoughts to be positive

Emotion provoking situation	'Accompanying thoughts and emotions'	'Positive thought replacement'
Reflecting on the injury	'When I think about the injury, I replay it in my mind and I get angry when I think about what happened'	'I will say to myself dwelling on the error won't help me recover – If I made an error then I will learn from that error but once the lesson is learned I will move on
'I get a sense of frustration when I see others go and train or compete'	'I am not progressing; it's not fair'	'I will focus on my rehabilitation programme – even when I am training I have recovery and rest days; let's see this day as one of them and something body needs'
'Doing rehabilitation exercisers that do not look strenuous to an onlooker'	'I feel silly doing these exercisers; I used to perform like an athlete and now I feel like a pensioner!'	'This is progress; I am getting closer to full fitness'
Your go. Pick a situation around injury	Write down your thoughts and emotions in this situation	Replace these thoughts with positive ones

Table 24.3 If-Then plans for injured athletes

If (barrier to performance)	Then (solution to the barrier)
If I notice I feel frustrated that I am not recovering fast enough …	Then I will take a deep breathe and focusing on the word relax as I breathe out and then I will say to myself … be patient!
If I feel the injury and I start thinking that I will never recover …	Then I will say to myself; no need to think that far ahead – just focus on doing the next thing!
If I think that they might be a miracle cure …	Then I will remind myself that the best thing to do is follow the rehab plan and if I do that then I have done a good job!

should be aware that the athlete's emotions might affect the severity of how the injury is presented, and that the doctor's feedback can influence athlete emotions. Encouraging athletes to use techniques to help shield unwanted inner states.

Summary

Injury is something that is highly likely to occur during an athletic career. Injuries can have major psychological consequences and unpleasant emotions and thoughts that occur once injured can prolong the recovery process. Helping athletes work through a process where they accept the injury can help manage unwanted inner states. The physician is a powerful source of feedback and encouraging the athletes to work on psychological states such as using emotion regulation strategies could have the dual benefit of improving adherence to rehabilitation programmes and improving the well-being of the athlete.

to do – in this way, the individual might use a technique such as imagery and see themselves perform the task successfully and thereby evoke feelings of self-confidence. The person could try to re-appraise the task so that it is not so important to complete. Alternatively, the individual could re-appraise the emotion, for example, see anxiety as a signal that the task is important or see depression as something to avoid and increase the intensity of effort in order to do so. The individual could also try to suppress the emotion; that is trying to reduce its intensity by ignoring it. However, suppression comes with a warning signal as it is a strategy has been found to be the least effective and associates with physiological markers of stress.

If-then plans have been found to be an effective method of changing thought processes (see Table 24.3). If-then plans work by putting the barrier to poor performance alongside the solution. By putting barriers and solutions side by side, the process of implementing the solution can become automated. During the learning stages, people repeat the if-then plan daily until it becomes ingrained. If-then plans can re-structure negative thoughts and turn them into positive thoughts by having pre-prepared structured statements (Table 24.3).

In summary, injury comes with negative psychological states including unpleasant moods and emotions. The medical team

Further reading

Devonport, T.J., Lane, A.M. & Hanin, Y. (2005) Emotional states of athletes prior to performance induced injury. *Journal of Sports Science & Medicine*, **4**, 382–394.

Lane, A. M., Beedie, C. J., Jones, M. V., Uphill, M., & Devonport, T. J. (2011). The BASES expert statement on emotion regulation in sport. *The Sport and Exercise Scientist*, **29**, 14-15. www.bases.org.uk/BASES-Expert-Statements

Lane, A.M., Beedie, C.J., Jones, M.V., Uphill, M. & Devonport, T.J. (2012) The BASES expert statement on emotion regulation in sport. *The Journal of Sport Sciences*, **30**, 1189–1195. doi:10.1080/02640414.2012.693621

Stevens, M. J., & Lane, A. M. (2001). Mood-regulating strategies used by athletes. *Athletic Insight*. http://www.athleticinsight.com/Vol3Iss3/MoodRegulation.htm

Terry, P.C., Lane, A.M. & Fogarty, G. (2003) Construct validity of the Profile of Mood States-A for use with adults. *Psychology of Sport and Exercise*, **4**, 125–139.

Webb, T.L., Miles, E., Sheeran, P., Gallo, I.S. & Gollwitzer, P.M. (2012) Effective regulation of affect: an action control perspective on emotion regulation. *European Review of Social Psychology*, **23** (**1**), 143–186.

Index

Notes: Page references in *italics* refers to figures, tables and boxed material.

ABCDE approach 9
abrasions, facial 21, *21*, 25
acclimatisation
    altitude 81–2
    heat 69, 71, *71*
acetazolamide 83, *84*, 85
Achilles tendinopathy *40*
aciclovir 50
active in later life
    definitions *102*
    disability prevention *102*, 102–4, *103*, *104*
    disease prevention and management 102
    exercise groups 106
    frailty prevention *102*, 102–4, *103*, *104*
    functional capacity, maintenance of 104
    immobility prevention *102*, 102–4, *103*, *104*
    isolation prevention 104
    medical referral responsibilities 107, *108*
    NICE recommendations 107, *107*
    providing guidance and opportunity 104–8
    safety 106–7, *107*
    types of activity 104–5, *105*
    UK physical activity guidelines 105–6, *106*
acute mountain sickness (AMS) *82*, 82–3, *83*
Advanced Trauma Life Support (ATLS)
    guidelines 17
American football 10, 16, 19
amoxicillin 43, 53
amphetamine 119
anabolic agents
    anabolic androgenic steroids 116–17, *117*
    clenbutarol 117
    peptide hormones 117–18
    zeranol 117
archery
    rate of injury and illness *1*
    summer sport *90*
arrhythmias 62, 72
articular osteochondrosis 35, *35*
athlete biological passport 120–121
athlete goals and emotions
    doctors influence on 123
    injury affects on 122–3

athlete's heart *see* heart, athlete's
athletes mood, injury presentation
    cognitive strategies 124–5
    confidence, lack of 124
    emotion regulation strategies 124, *124*
    frustration 124
    goal-setting process 124
    if-then plans 125, *125*
    mood state scale 123, *123*
    normal athlete *vs.* injured athlete 123, *124*
    unpleasant moods and emotions 125
ATMIST handover 8
ATP 111, *113*, 114
azithromycin 53

bacterial skin infections 50–51, *51*
badminton, rate of injury and illness *1*
basal metabolic rate 110
benignpositional paroxysmal vertigo (BPPV)
    11
β-2 agonists 45, 48, 117, 118, *118*
beta-alanine 114
bicarbonate loading 114, *114*
black eye 27
blood transfusion 119, *119*
blood-borne viruses 52, *52*
body
    cold *see* cold
    heat influence on *see* heat
    temperature 67–8
bone mineral density (BMD) 59
boxing
    head injury 10
    rate of injury and illness *1*
breath-hold diving 76, 77
brisk exercise 93
bronchodilator challenge test 45, *46*
bronchoprovocation testing 45, *45*
burnout *see* unexplained underperformance
    syndrome (overtraining syndrome)

caffeine 114–15
cannabinoids 120

carbohydrate 109–10
    dehydration solutions 113
    loading 113
    metabolism 111
    post-exercise consumption 113
carnitine 114
cefuroxime axetil 53
chemical manipulation prohibition 119
childhood injury management
    child protection 32–3, *33*
    hip pathology 36, 36–7
    malignancy 37
    non-accidental injury red flags 32, *33*
    overuse skeletal injuries *see* osteochondrosis in
        children
    physiological changes 32, *32*
    physical growth 31, 31–2, *32*
    psychological 32
    skeletal injuries, acute
        buckle fractures/torus fractures 33, *33*
        greenstick fractures 33
        physeal injuries 33, *34*
        tendon-bone junctions 33, *33*
childhood obesity 94
chloramphenicol eye ointment 43
choroidal ruptures 28, *28*
chronic fatigue syndrome
    in athletes *see* unexplained underperformance
        syndrome (overtraining syndrome)
    causes 55
chronic traumatic encephalopathy (CTE) 10,
    19–20
ciprofloxacin 42
clarithromycin 51
clenbutarol 117
climbers, snow blindness 28
clindamycin 51
clothing
    cold environment 73
    heat environment 71
codeine (pain killer) 43
cold environment
    acclimatisation 73

ABC of Sports and Exercise Medicine, Fourth Edition.
Edited by Gregory P. Whyte, Mike Loosemore and Clyde Williams.
© 2015 John Wiley & Sons, Ltd. Published 2015 by John Wiley & Sons, Ltd.

cold environment (*continued*)
  clothing 73
  injuries
    freezing (frostbite) 74, *74*
    non-freezing cold injury 74, *74*
    risk assessment 75, *75*
  performance effects 72, *72–3*
cold sensitivity 74
cold water immersion 72
commotio retinae 27, *28*
computed tomography
  blowout fracture 24, *24*
  traumatic brain injury 19, *19*
concussion
  definition 10
  pathophysiology 11, 16, *16*, *17*
  return-to-play 19
  symptoms and signs 10–11, *11*
consciousness loss 10
contact lenses 29
corticotrophins 118

darbepoietin 117, 118
decompression illness 78, *79*
dehydration
  carbohydrate and electrolyte solutions 113
  in cold environments 73
  heat 69
  prevention 113
dengue fever 42
dental injury 22, *22*, 25
dexamethasone 83, 85
diabetes
  cumulative incidence of 96
  obesity, risk factor for 96
diarrhoeal illness 50
disability in sports
  anti-doping considerations 91
  choosing a sport/activity 90–91, *91*
  injury risk 91
  medical education and training 91
  paralympic sports *see* paralympic sports
diuretics 119
diving
  amateur scuba diving 78–9
  barotrauma 78
  breath hold diving 77
  decompression illness 78, *79*
  immersion effects
    cooling 76
    hydrostatic effects 76, *77*
  pressure effects 76–7
  rate of injury and illness *1*
  scuba diving *see* scuba diving
dizziness 11
doxycycline 53
drugs in sport
  anabolic agents *see* anabolic agents
  athlete biological passport 120–121
  cannabinoids 120
  glucocorticosteriods 120
  narcotics 120
  prohibited methods
    in-and out-of-competition 119
    in-competition 119–20
  prohibited substances
    in-and out-of-competition 116–19

in-competition 119–20
dual X-ray absorptiometry (DXA) 59

ear stones 11
education, eye injury prevention 26
elderly. *see* active in later life
electrocardiograms 62, *63*
elite young athletes
  aerobic fitness 99, *99*, *100*
  growth and maturation 97–8
  muscle strength 98, *98–9*, *99*
  physical characteristics 97, *98*
emergency action plan 5, *5*
emergency medical management in individual and
    team sports *5*
energy metabolism 111
energy balance *110*, 110–111, *111*
energy expenditure 60, 86, 94–6, 110, 111, 115,
    120
energy intake 110, *110*
environmental factors
  altitude *see* high altitude
  cold *see* cold environment
  heat *see* heat
  temperature 67–8
ephedrine 119
epidemiological studies of sports injuries and
    illnesses
  classification 2, *2*
  definition 2, *2*
  examples of *2*
  rate of 2–3, *3*
  risk factors 3, *3*
  severity 3, *3*
  study design and population 1–2
equipment
  immediate care 9
  for scuba diving 76, *76*
ergogenic supplements
  beta-alanine 114
  bicarbonate loading 114, *114*
  caffeine 114–15
  carnitine 114
  creatine *113*, 113–14, *114*
  nitrates 113
  nutritional supplements 113
erythema chronicum migrans (ECM) rash 52, *52*
erythromycin 51
erythropoiesis-stimulating agents
    (ESAs) 117–18, *118*
erythropoietin (EPO) 117–18
erythropoietin gene doping 119
essential amino acid supplements 110
eucapnic voluntary hyperpnoea (EVH) challenge
    test 46, 47, *47*
European Society of Cardiology (ESC) 62
exercise
  for angina 86
  continuous and interval-type training 87–8
  historical example of 86
  intensities for aerobic 87, *88*
  training 87–8
exercise challenge test 46–7
exercise-induced asthma (EIA) 45, *45*
exercise-induced bronchoconstriction (EIB)
  differential diagnosis 48–9, *49*
  diagnosis of

bronchodilator challenge 45, *46*
  follow-up assessments 47
  indirect airway challenges *see* Indirect airway
      challenges
  objective support 47
  vs. EILO 49
  management strategies 47, *48*
  prevalence *44*, 45
  screening for 47
  treatment
    non-pharmacological interventions 47
    pharmacological interventions 48
exercise-induced laryngeal obstruction
    (EILO) 49
eye injuries
  assessment 29, *29*
  blowout fractures 27, *27*, *28*
  burns 28
  choroidal ruptures 28, *28*
  commotio retinae 27, *28*
  corneal abrasion 27, *27*
  first aid 29, *29*
  foreign particles 28
  globe ruptures 28
  hyphaema 27, *28*
  intraocular blunt trauma 27–8
  penetrating injuries 28, *28*
  periorbital contusionor (blackeye) 27
  prevention and protection 26, *27*
  retinal tear 27
  retro-bulbar haemorrhage 27
  sports associated with 26
  subconjunctival haemorrhage 27
  superficial blunt trauma 27
  visual correction methods 29–30, *30*
  vitreous haemorrhage 27

facial and jaw injuries *see also* eye injuries
  dental injury 22, *22*
  internal orbital (blow out) fractures 23–4, *24*
  mandibular fractures 24, *24*
  maxillofacial fractures 22, *22*, 23
  middle-third facial fractures 24–5, *25*
  nasal fractures 22–3
  soft tissue injuries
    abrasions 21, *21*, 25
    haematomas 21
    lacerations 21–2, *22*
  treatment 24
  zygomatic (cheekbone) fractures 23, *23*, *24*
fat
  consumption 110
  metabolism 111
  storage 111
Fat Camps 95
female athlete triad
  bone health 59
  definition 58
  eating disorders 59
  health consequences 59
  low-energy availability 58
  menstrual function *58*, 58–9
  menstrual health 59
  prevention 58, 60
  screening and diagnosis
    annual screening questionnaire 59
    blood investigations 59, *60*

DXA scanning 60
treatment 60
flucloxacillin 51
football
    eye injury risk 26
    mature athlete retirement age 38
    rate of injury and illness *1*
    summer sport *90*
fractures
    blowout
        eye injuries 27, *27, 28*
        facial and jaw injuries 23–4, *24*
    buckle/torus, in children 33, *33*
    greenstick, in children 33
    Le Fort classification 25, *25*
    mandibular 24, *24*
    maxillofacial 22, *22, 23*
    middle-third facial 24–5, *25*
    nasal 22–3
    Salter-Harris classification 33–4, *34*
    stress *see* stress fractures
    zygomatic (cheekbone) 23, *23, 24*
freezing injury (frostbite) 74, *74*
functional overreaching 54
fungal skin infections 50

gas embolism 78, *79*
gene doping 119
geriatric obesity 94
Glasgow Coma Scale (GCS) 7, 17
globe ruptures 28
glycaemic index *110*
glycogenolysis 111
growth hormone (rhGH) 118, *118*
gymnastics 35, 60, 97–8

haematoma
    extradural 17, *17*
    facial injuries 21
    nasal septal 21
    subperichondrial 21
hamstring strain *40–41*
hard lenses, eye injuries 29
Head Impact Telemetry (HIT) 20
head injuries
    chronic traumatic encephalopathy 19
    concussion *see* concussion
    epidemiology 10
    management 17–19
    neurosurgical head injury 17, *18*
    pathophysiology 11, 16, *16, 17*
    prevention 20
    second impact syndrome 17
    types of 10–16, *11–16*
headache 10, 11, 17, 53, 69, 82, 83, 84
heart, athlete's
    cardiomyopathy 64–5, *65*
    cardiovascular adaptation to exercise 64, *64*
    ECG 62, *63*
    echocardiographic changes 62, 64
    emergency medical care 66
    pre-participation screening in young
        athlete 65–6, *66*
    repolarisation changes in black athletes 62
    sudden cardiac death 64, *65*
heat
    acclimatisation 71, *71*

body cooling 70
clothing *71*
dehydration during exercise 69
evaporation of sweat *68*
exertional rhabdomyolysis *69*
fluid balance maintenance 69–70
illness 69, *69*
    performance effects 68
    prescriptive zone 68, *68*
    psychological skills training 71
    risk assessment *71*
heat cramps 69
heat exhaustion 69
heat illness 69, *69*
heat stroke 69
helmets
    head injury, prevention of 19–20
    removal in concussion injuries 18
Hemopure 119
hepatitis 52
herpes gladiatorum 50
herpes simplex viruses 50, *51*
high altitude
    acclimatisation 81–2
    altitude-related disorder, medical
        management 84, *84*
    athlete at 84–5
    central nervous system *84*
    corneal thickening *84*
    cough *84*
    description 81, *82*
    environment physiologically challenging 81, *81*
    gastrointestinal upset *84*
    illnesses 82
    retinal haemorrhages *84*
    sleep disorder *84*
    thromboembolic disease *84*
high-altitude cerebral oedema (HACE) 83, *83*
high-altitude pulmonary oedema (HAPE)
    case study 83
    incidence 83–4
    pathophysiology 84
    treatment 84
hip osteochondritis dissecans 36–7
hockey
    ice 20, 101
    rate of injury and illness *1*
    underwater 76
hormone modulators 118–19
human immunodeficiency virus (HIV) 52
hyphaema 27, *28*
hyponatraemia *70*
hypothermia 72, 73, *73*, 76, 78, 79, 82
hypovolaemia 32

ibuprofen 43, 83
imidazole antifungal creams 50
immediate care
    emergency action plan 5, *5*
    initial assessment and management
        definitive care 8
        primary survey *see* primary survey of
            patient
        re-evaluation 7
        resuscitation 7
        safe approach 6, *6*

    secondary survey 7–8, *8*
    medical emergencies 9
    medical equipment 9
    musculoskeletal trauma 8
    spinal injury 8, *8*
    in sport 5
    wound care 9
immediate medical management on the field of
    play 5
immobility prevention in later life *102*, 102–4, *103, 104*
incisional surgery 29, *30*
indirect airway challenges test
    EVH challenge test *46, 47, 47*
    exercise challenge test 46–7
    expected flow-volume response *46*
    mannitol challenge test 47, *48*
infections
    bacterial skin 50–51, *51*
    fungal skin 50
    hepatitis 52
    herpes simplex viruses 50, *51*
    HIV 52
    leptospirosis 53, *53*
    lyme disease *52*, 52–3
    pityriasis versicolor 50
    tinea corporis 50
    tinea pedis (athlete's foot) 50
    upper respiratory tract 52
    viral skin 50, *51*
    warts (verrucas) 50
infectious mononucleosis 52
infraorbital nerve injury 23, *23*
inhaled asthma medication 48
injury and illness
    classification 2, *2*
    definition 2, *2*
    rate of *1*, 2–3, *3*
    risk factors 3, *3*
    severity 3, *3*
insulin 118, 119
insulin-likegrowth factor (IGF-1) 59, 117, 118
International Olympic Committee 45, 65
    aerobic fitness enhancement *99*
    caffeine ban (lifted) 115
intra-corneal LASIK 29
intraoral laceration 22, *22*, 25
iron
    deficiency anaemia 113
    overload 117
    stores, unexplained underperformance
        syndrome 56
Isotope Ratio Mass Spectrometry (IRMS) 121

jaw injuries *see* facial and jaw injuries
judo
    rate of injury and illness *1*
    summer sport *90*

ketoconazole shampoo 50
knee osteoarthritis *40*

lacerations, facial 21–2, *22*
lactate 114
lactic acid 111
Le Fort fracture classification 25, *25*
Leptospira 53
leptospirosis 53, *53*

'les autres' *90*
limb injuries 8, *8*
liver glycogen 111
locorten vioform 43
long-term metabolites (LTMs) 117
loperamide 42, 43
lucid interval, extradural haemotomas 17
lyme disease *52*, 52–3

macronutrients 109–10, *110*
Maddocks questions 12–15, 19
magnetic resonance imaging, traumatic brain
    injury 19, *19*
malaria 41
management in children *see* childhood injury
    management
mandibular fractures 24, *24*
mannitol challenge test 47, *48*
mature athlete
    definition 38
    musculoskeletal injuries in *see* musculoskeletal
        injuries
maxillofacial fractures 22, *22*, *23 see also specific
    types*
medical cardiac and pitch-side skills 5
medical care, major sport events
    athlete village
        covering venues 43
        doping 43
        equipment 43
        local language 43
        media training 43
        medical provision 42–3
        medical room availability 42
        medical team selection 43
    at event
        dog bites 42
        food 42
        snake bites 42
        weather condition 42
        Weil's disease, rats causes 42
    medical records collection 41
    before travelling
        adaption to altitude 42
        anti-malarial medication 41
        immunisations 41
        insect repellants 42
        long-sleeved clothes 42
        mosquito bites, prevention from 41
    during travelling
        jet lag effect 42
        medicines 43
        mode of transport 42
        travel sickness 42
    up-to-date therapeutic use exemption form 41
menstrual cycle, healthy 60
menstrual disorders, female athlete triad *58*,
    58–9
metformin 96
methylephedrine 119
methylhexaneamine 119
microdosing 118
micronutrients 110
middle-third facial fractures 24–5, *25*
mineral supplements 110
mixed gas diving 78
mountain sickness, acute *82*, 82–3, *83*

mouth guards
    concussion prevention 20
    dental injury prevention 22
mupirocin ointment 51
musculoskeletal injuries
    age factors 38
    case scenario *39*, *40*
    contributing factors 39, *39*
    injury prevention 38
    management 39, 39–40
musculoskeletal trauma 8, *8*
myocarditis, viral 56
myostatin inhibitors 118–19

nandrolone 116
narcotics 120
National Institute for Health and Care Excellence
    (NICE) 96
negative energy balance 58, 111
nifedipine 83, 84
nitrates 113
nitric oxide 47, 113
nitrogen, diving 77, 78, 79
nitrogen narcosis 77, 78, 79
nitrox, scuba diving 78
non-approved substances 116
non-articular osteochondrosis 35, *35*
non-freezing cold injury 74, *74*
non-functional overreaching 54
non-steroidal anti-inflammatory drugs 43
nordic walking *103*
nose
    fractures 22–3
    septal haematomas 21
nutrition
    macronutrients 109–10, *110*
    micronutrients 110
    role 109
    strategies
        after exercise 113
        before exercise 111–13
        during exercise 113
nutritional supplements 113

obesity
    appetite and 95
    built environment and 96
    and physical activity
        childhood 94
        vs. diet, control of 94–5
        fat reduction 95, *96*
        geriatric obesity 94
        guidelines 93–4
        lifestyle and 96
        microactivity 96
        moderate intensity, examples 95, *96*
        and mortality 94
        significant health benefits 95, *95*
        weight reduction 95
oligomenorrhoea 58
open fractures 8
Osgood-Schlatter's disease *34*
osteoarthritis, knee *40*
osteochondrosis in children
    articular 35, *35*
    non-articular 35, *35*
    spinal physeal 35

osteoporosis 58, 59, 102
over reaching 55, 56
overhydration *70*
overtraining syndrome *see* unexplained
    underperformance syndrome (overtraining
    syndrome)
overuse injuries
    in children 34–6, *35*, *36*
oxygen
    maximum consumption *see* VO$_{2max}$
    partial pressures of 77, 79
    scuba diving 78

Panner's disease 35
Panton–Valentine leucocidin (PVL) toxin 51, *51*
paracetamol 43, 83
paralympic sports
    changing perceptions *92*
    classification 90
    eligible impairment types 90, *90*
    medical impairment types 90, *90*
    summer sports, list of *90*, *91*
    winter sports 90
participation risk, disability in sport 91
pars intra-articularis, stress fractures 35, *36*
penetrating eye injuries 28, *28*
penicillin 42, 43, 53
peptide hormones 117
perfluorocarbons 119
periorbital contusion (black eye) 27
Perthes, in children 36
phosphocreatine 99, 111, 113, *113*
physical activity *see also* exercise
    ABC elements 86
    childhood 94
    vs. diet, control of 94–5
    geriatric obesity 94
    guidelines 93–4
    historical examples 86
    in later life *see* active in later life
    lifestyle and 96
    microactivity 96
    and mortality 94
    risk reduction 87, *87*
    waking hours spent levels 86–7, *87*
physical inactivity 86
physical incapacitation of cold water
    immersion 72
physical manipulation prohibition 119
physician
    feedback on injured athlete's *see* psychological
        states of injured athlete
    team 82, 85
pistol shooting, disabled athletes 91
Plasmodium parasites 41
pneumothorax, barotrauma 78
post-concussion headache 11
prescriptive zone, temperature 68, *68*
prevalence of EIB *44*, *45*
prevalence of illness 3, *3*
prevention
    cervical spine injury 6, *6*
    concussion 20
    dehydration 113
    dental injury, mouth guards 22
    disability in later life *102*, 102–4, *103*, *104*
    disease in later life 102

female athlete triad 60
frailty in later life *102*, 102–4, *103*, *104*
immobility in later life *102*, 102–4, *103*, *104*
injury 38
isolation in later life 104
unexplained underperformance
    syndrome 56–7, *57*
primary survey of patient
    airway maintenance with c-spine protection 6,
        6
    breathing assessment 6–7
    catastrophic bleeding management 6
    circulation assessment 7, *7*
    exposure and environment control 7
    neurological assessment 7, *7*
protective eyewear 26
protein consumption 110
pseudoephedrine 119, 120
psychological skills training (PST) 71
psychological states of injured athlete
    doctors influence 123
    goals and emotions, affects on 122–3, *123*
    Kublar–Ross model *123*
    moods influence *see* athletes mood, injury
        presentation
pulmonary barotrauma 78, 79
pulmonary dysfunction in athletes
    EIB, assessment and management *see*
        exercise-induced bronchoconstriction
        (EIB)
    physiology 44
    symptoms 44, *44*
pulmonary oedema 76, *77*, 79
puncture wounds, facial 21

rabies vaccine 42
radiograph
    articular osteochondrosis 35
    endochondral ossification 31, *32*
    zygomatic (cheekbone) fractures 42
recombinant human erythropoietin 117–18
refractive surgery 29–30, *30*
Register of Exercise Professionals 107
resuscitation and emergency aid 5
Retinal tear 27
rewarming of freezing injury 74
rhabdomyolysis, exertional 69
road racing, wheelchair 91
rowing
    rate of injury and illness *1*
    summer sport *90*
rugby union/league
    herpes simplex virus 50
    international, injury incidence *3*
    stress fracture 35
running
    distance, daily food intake *109*
    long-distance 64
    weight loss for competition 109

safety
    active in later life 106–7, *107*
    approach for injured athlete 6, *6*
sailing
    rate of injury and illness *1*
    summer sport *90*
salbutamol 45, 118

salmeterol 84, 118
Salter–Harris classification of fractures 33–4,
    34
scrumpox 50, *51*
scuba diving
    air 77, *78*
    amateur 78–9
    equipment for 76, *76*
    mixed gas diving 78
    nitrox 78
    oxygen 78
second impact syndrome 17
secondary survey, immediate care 7, *8*
sedentary behaviour
    definition 104, *104*
    effect in old age 104, *104*
selective androgen receptor modulators
    (SARMs) 117
selenium sulphide shampoo 50
septic arthritis, in children 36
severity of injury measurement 3
shivering 67, 72, 73
shooting
    disabled athletes 91
    rate of injury and illness *1*
    spectacles 29
skeletal muscle, glycogen content 111, *112*
skiing 19, 75, 90
skin and soft tissue infections
    bacterial skin infections
        impetigo 50–51
        S. aureus and PVL toxin 51, *51*
    fungal skin infections 50
    viral skin infections 50, *51*
skin bends (cutaneous decompression illness)
    79
slipped femoral epiphysis, in children 36
snow blindness 28
socialisation opportunities in elderly 104
soft lenses 29
soft tissue injuries, facial *see* facial and jaw
    injuries
spectacles, eye injuries 29
spinal injury 8, *8*
spinal physeal injuries in children 35
spinal vertebra stress fracture 35, *36*
spirometry 46, *47*
spondylolisthesis 36
spondylolysis 36
sport events, medical care *see* medical care, major
    sport events
sport participation
    changes in *89*
    educational toolkit topics *89*
    and resources *89*
sports drinks 113
sports fatigue syndrome *see* unexplained
    underperformance syndrome (overtraining
    syndrome)
sprint racing, wheelchair 91
sprinting 111, 114
standard principles of resuscitation and trauma
    immediate care 5
staphylococcal infection 50–51, *51*
Staphylococcus aureus 50, 51
stimulants 119–20
Streptococcus pyogenes 50

stress fractures
    female athlete triad 59
    management 36
    pars intra-articularis 35, *36*
    of tibia in child 36
stresses (non-sports related) 54, 55
study design, epidemiological 1–2
study population 1–2
subconjunctival haemorrhage 27, *28*
subluxation of teeth 22
subperichondrial haematoma 21
sudden cardiac death 64, *65*
surface-based laser surgery 29
sweat 68, 70, 71
sweat glands 68
sweat suits 71
swimming
    to burn off fat 95
    disabled athletes 91
    elderly 105
    rate of injury and illness *1*
    relative age effect 101
Symptom Evaluation section of the Sports
    Concussion Assessment Tool (SCAT3) 11,
    12–15
systematic approach 6, *6*

table tennis
    moderate intensity physical activity 96
    rate of injury and illness *1*
    summer sport *90*
target population epidemiological studies 2
teeth injury 22, *22*
tendon bone junction injuries in children
    acute 33, *33*
    overuse injuries 35
tennis
    boys early maturity benefits 98
    rate of injury and illness *1*
    relative age effect 101
tension pneumothorax 78
terbutaline 118
testosterone 119, 121
tetanus immunisation 41
tetracosactrin 118
tetrahydrogestrinone (THG) 117
Therapeutic Use Exemption (TUE) certificate
    116
thermal balance 67
thermic effect of exercise 110
thermoregulatory system 67, 68
Tour de France, illegal drug use 116
trace elements, unexplained underperformance
    syndrome 56
tramadol 116, 120
travel associated infections
    malaria 41
    travellers' diarrhea 42
travel, medical care
    adaption to altitude 42
    anti-malarial medication 41
    immunisations 41
    insect repellants 42
    jet lag effect 42
    long-sleeved clothes 42
    medicines 43
    mode of transport 42

travel, medical care (*continued*)
    mosquito bites, prevention from 41
    travel sickness 42
triathlon
    death due to cold effect 72
    rate of injury and illness *1*
triglycerides 110, 111
type 2 diabetes 94, 96

unconsciousness
    breath-hold diving 77
    high-altitude cerebral oedema 83
    scuba diving 77
    in unprotected airway 6
under-recovery syndrome *see* unexplained
    underperformance syndrome (overtraining
    syndrome)
underwater hockey 76
underwater orienteering 76
unexplained underperformance syndrome
    (overtraining syndrome) 100, *100*
    definition 54
    diet 56
    early detection 56, *57*
    heart rate 56
    immune suppression by *55*
    investigation
        full blood count 56
        hormonal assessment 56
        iron stores 56
        laboratory tests 56
        trace elements 56
        viruses 56
        vitamins 56
    management 57, *57*

precipitating factors 54, *54*
prevention 56
signs 55
stages of 54, *54*
stressors 55
symptoms 54–5, *55*
training history 55, *55*
United States Anti-Doping Agency (USADA)
    116
upper limb problems, disabled athletes
    participation risk 91
upper respiratory tract infections 52
urine sample testing 117

ventricular arrhythmias 64
ventricular cavity sizes, right and left 64
ventricular wall thickness, left 62, 64, 65, *65*
verrucas 50
viral haemorrhagic fever *see* dengue fever
viruses
    blood-borne 52
    infections 50, *51*
    unexplained underperformance syndrome 56
visually impaired 91
vital signs 6, 7
vitamin C 56
vitamin D 60
vitamin K 60
vitamins
    micronutrient 110
    unexplained underperformance syndrome 56
vitreous haemorrhage 27
volleyball, rate of injury and illness *1*
VO_{2max}
    altitude effect 84

cold water immersion effect 72–3
energy metabolism 111
exercise intensity monitoring 86–7
in hot climates 68
vasoconstrictor effect 119

walking
    brisk 94, 95, *96*
    easy, light activity 86, *87*
    nordic *103*
warm down 70
warm up 38, 47, 106
warts (verrucas) 50
weight loss
    for competition 109
    exercise 95, *95*, *96*
Weil's disease 42
wheelchair
    basketball 91
    road racing 91
    sprint racing 91
    wheeling, benefits 93, 95
wind chill *75*
Wingate anaerobic test 100
World Anti-Doping Agency (WADA) 48, 85, 116,
    119, 120
World Anti-Doping Code 91
wounds, immediate care 9
wrestling
    herpes simplex virus 50, *51*
    rate of injury and illness *1*
wrist radiograph *34*

zeranol 117
zygomatic (cheekbone) fractures 23, *23*, *24*